Cartilage and Bone Development and Its Disorders

Endocrine Development

Vol. 21

Series Editor

P.-E. Mullis Bern

4th ESPE Advanced Seminar in Developmental Endocrinology, Stockholm, June 30–July 1, 2010

Cartilage and Bone Development and Its Disorders

Volume Editors

Cecilia Camacho-Hübner Stockholm/New York, N.Y.
Ola Nilsson Stockholm
Lars Sävendahl Stockholm

20 figures and 3 tables, 2011

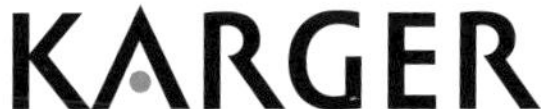

Basel · Freiburg · Paris · London · New York · New Delhi · Bangkok · Beijing · Tokyo · Kuala Lumpur · Singapore · Sydney

Endocrine Development

Founded 1999 by Martin O. Savage, London

Cecilia Camacho-Hübner
Division of Pediatric Endocrinology
Department of Women´s and Children's Health
Karolinska Institutet and University Hospital
Stockholm, Sweden

Ola Nilsson
Center for Molecular Medicine and
Division of Pediatric Endocrinology
Department of Women's and Children's Health
Karolinska Institutet and University Hospital
Stockholm, Sweden

Lars Sävendahl
Division of Pediatric Endocrinology
Department of Women's and Children's Health
Karolinska Institutet and University Hospital
Stockholm, Sweden

Library of Congress Cataloging-in-Publication Data

ESPE Advanced Seminar in Developmental Endocrinology (4th : 2010 : Stockholm, Sweden)
Cartilage and bone development and its disorders / 4th ESPE Advanced Seminar in Developmental Endocrinology, Stockholm, June 30-July 1, 2010 ; volume editors, Cecilia Camacho-Hübner, Ola Nilsson, Lars Sävendahl.
p. ; cm. -- (Endocrine development, ISSN 1421-7082 ; v. 21)
Includes bibliographical references and index.
ISBN 978-3-8055-9792-0 (hard cover : alk. paper) -- ISBN 978-3-8055-9793-7 (e-ISBN)
1. Bone diseases in children--Congresses. 2. Bones--Growth--Congresses. 3. Pediatric endocrinology--Congresses. 4. Cartilage--Diseases--Congresses. 5. Cartilage--Growth--Congresses. 6. Chondrogenesis--Congresses. I. Camacho-Hübner, Cecilia. II. Nilsson, Ola. III. Sävendahl, Lars. IV. Title. V. Series: Endocrine development ; v. 21. 1421-7082
[DNLM: 1. Cartilage--growth & development--Congresses. 2. Bone Development--genetics--Congresses. 3. Bone Diseases, Endocrine--Congresses. 4. Cartilage Diseases--Congresses. W1 EN3635 v.21 2011 / WE 300]
RJ482.B65E87 2010
618.92'71--dc23

2011020217

Bibliographic Indices. This publication is listed in bibliographic services, including Current Contents® and PubMed/MEDLINE.

www.karger.com
Printed in Switzerland on acid-free and non-aging paper (ISO 9706) by Reinhardt Druck, Basel
ISSN 1421–7082
ISBN 978–3–8055–9792–0
e-ISBN 978–3–8055–9793–7

Contents

Acknowledgments

The Scientific Organizing Committee on behalf of the European Society for Paediatric Endocrinology (ESPE) takes this opportunity to thank the Department of Women's and Children's Health at Karolinska Institutet and Astrid Lindgren Children's Hospital, Stockholm, for facilitation of this educational event.

Special thanks go to ESPE and Ipsen for their generous sponsorship of the 4th Advanced Seminar in Developmental Endocrinology and to all researchers for their contributions to the present book.

Preface

Childhood growth is severely impaired in endocrine and other systemic childhood diseases, including cancer, gastrointestinal, pulmonary, and cardiac disorders. In addition, over 300 different genetic diseases directly inhibit the ability of the growth plate to form new bone, leaving affected children with growth failure and bony deformities that can severely impact their quality of life and general health and sometimes lead to early death. In order to find new treatments, we first need to understand these diseases and how normal bone growth and metabolism are accomplished.

The purpose of the European Society for Paediatric Endocrinology (ESPE) Advanced Seminars is to convene researchers and pediatric endocrinologists to facilitate exchange of knowledge, ideas and recent findings, and thereby advance translational research in selected areas of developmental endocrinology. At the 4th Seminar, there were 12 invited presentations on selected topics in the field of cartilage and bone development and diseases. The lectures covered areas stretching from the local regulation of growth plate cartilage to new perspectives on the use of stem cells and cartilage tissue engineering. The program also included a workshop addressing methodologies essential for the progress of this research field. In addition, 10 young investigators gave oral presentations highlighting their recent data. Three of these were awarded a prize for outstanding scientific contribution to the field.

This series of *Developmental Endocrinology* has served as a forum for exchange of information providing a unique opportunity for researchers from various disciplines to contribute to our understanding of the field of cartilage and bone development and highlight important areas for future research.

All the chapters included in this issue have been written by international experts in their respective areas, and we are most grateful for their contributions.

Much progress has been made in the field, but there is still a long way to go to fully understand the pathogenesis of cartilage and bone disorders and their clinical presentation. Research that will bring new insights for the development of novel therapeutic strategies is therefore highly warranted.

Cecilia Camacho-Hübner, Stockholm/New York, N.Y.
Ola Nilsson, Stockholm
Lars Sävendahl, Stockholm

List of Abbreviations

ACFD	Acrocapitofemoral dysplasia
ACI	Autologous chondrocyte implantation
ACTH	Adrenocorticotropic hormone
ALP	Alkaline phosphatase
ALS	Acid-labile subunit
ARHR	Autosomal recessive hypophosphatemic rickets
ATF	Activating transcription factor
BDA1	Brachydactyly type A1
BERKO	Mouse strain deficient in ERβ
BMP	Bone morphogenetic protein
BNP	Brain natriuretic peptide
CDK	Cyclin-dependent kinase
CNP	C-type natriuretic peptide
COMP	Cartilage oligomeric matrix protein
CP	Columnar proliferating
CREB	cAMP response element-binding protein
C_t	Cycle threshold
DERKO	Mouse strains deficient in ERα and ERβ
E2	Estradiol
ECM	Extracellular matrix
ER	Estrogen receptor
ERα	Estrogen receptor-α
ERβ	Estrogen receptor-β
ERE	Estrogen-responsive element
ERKO	Mouse strain deficient in ERα
FD	Fibrous dysplasia
FGD	Familial (isolated) glucocorticoid deficiency
FGF	Fibroblast growth factor
FGFR	Fibroblast growth factor receptor
GACI	Generalized arterial calcification
GH	Growth hormone

GHBP	Growth hormone-binding protein
GHR	Growth hormone receptor
GHRH	Growth hormone-releasing hormone
GNAS1	Guanine nucleotide-binding protein, α-stimulating
GRP 30	G protein-coupled receptor 30
huCYC	Human cyclophilin
HZ	Hypertrophic zone
IGF1R	Insulin-like growth factor 1 receptor
IGFBP-3	Insulin-like growth factor binding protein
IGF-I	Insulin-like growth factor I
IHC	Immunohistochemistry
IHH	Indian hedgehog
IL-2	Interleukin-2
MAP	Mitogen-activated kinase
MED	Multiple epiphyseal dysplasia
MEF2c	Myocyte enhancer factor 2c
MEPE	Matrix extracellular phosphoglycoprotein
MF	Microfracture
MMP	Matrix metalloproteinase
MRAP	Melanocortin 2 receptor accessory protein
MSC	Mesenchymal stromal cell
OI	Osteogenesis imperfecta
OPG	Osteoprotegerin
PFD	Polyostotic fibrous dysplasia
PHEX	Phosphate-regulating endopeptidase homolog, X linked
Pi	Plasma phosphorus
PPR1	PTH/PTHrP receptor
PTH	Parathyroid hormone
PTHrP	Parathyroid hormone-related protein
PZ	Proliferative zone
rMED	Recessive multiple epiphyseal dysplasia
RNAi	RNA interference
RP	Round proliferating
RZ	Resting zone
SERM	Selective estrogen receptor modulator
siRNA	Small interfering RNA
STC1	Stanniocalcin 1
TGF-β	Transforming growth factor-β
THRB	Thyroid hormone receptor-β
TRPV5	Transient receptor potential V5

TUNEL	Terminal deoxynucleotidyl transferase-mediated deoxy-UTP nick-end labeling
VEGF	Vascular endothelial growth factor
XLHR	X-linked hypophosphatemic rickets

Camacho-Hübner C, Nilsson O, Sävendahl L (eds): Cartilage and Bone Development and Its Disorders.
Endocr Dev. Basel, Karger, 2011, vol 21, pp 1–11

Chondrocyte Proliferation and Differentiation

Manuela Wuelling · Andrea Vortkamp

Center for Medical Biotechnology, Department of Developmental Biology, University Duisburg-Essen, Essen, Germany

Abstract

The skeletal elements of the axial and appendicular skeleton are preformed as cartilage templates by a mechanism called endochondral ossification. During this process, a cartilage template is formed in which chondrocytes proliferate and differentiate into hypertrophic chondrocytes and are gradually replaced by bone. Postnatally, remnants of embryonic chondrocytes remain in a restricted domain between the ossified regions of the bones forming the growth plate. The coordinated proliferation and differentiation of chondrocytes ensures the continuous elongation of the epiphyseal growth plates. The sequential changes between proliferation and differentiation are tightly regulated by secreted growth factors, which activate chondrocyte-specific transcription factors. Transcription factors that play critical roles in regulating cell type-specific gene expression include SOX9, GLI2/3 and RUNX2. This review will outline recent advances in the analysis of the complex transcriptional network that regulates distinct steps of chondrocyte differentiation.

Endochondral Ossification

During endochondral ossification, bones are formed by two processes. During intramembranous ossification, by which the bones of the skull and part of the facial bones and clavicle are formed, mesenchymal cells directly differentiate into osteoblasts. In contrast, the axial and appendicular skeleton of vertebrates develops by endochondral ossification. During this process, the initial anlagen are formed as cartilage templates, which model the skeletal elements. Gradually, the cartilage templates are replaced by bone. The process of endochondral ossification starts with the condensation of mesenchymal cells, which differentiate into chondrocytes (fig. 1a, b). These cells initially proliferate and differentiate into two subpopulations of proliferating chondrocytes: round, low proliferating chondrocytes at the distal ends of the condensation (RP chondrocytes) and high proliferating chondrocytes that are organized

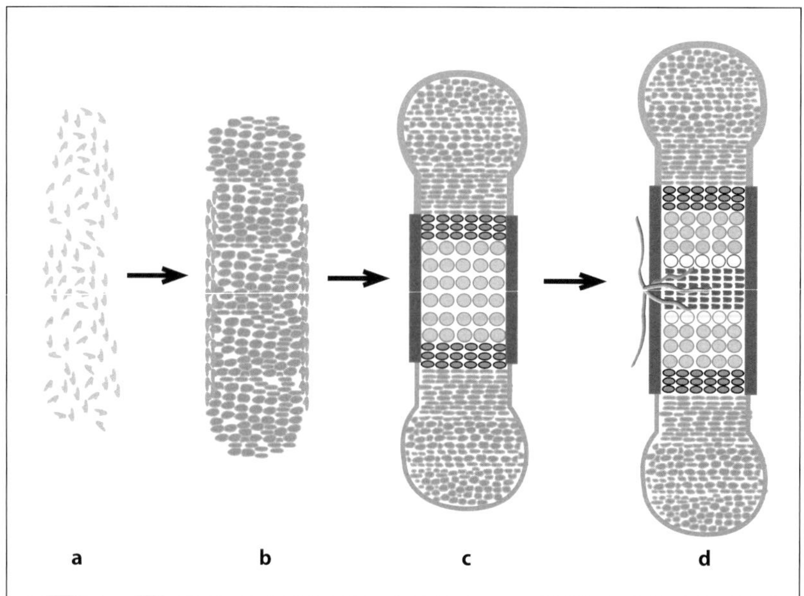

Fig. 1. Endochondral ossification requires sequential differentiation and degradation of chondrocytes. Mesenchymal cells condense to form the cartilage anlagen (**a**) and differentiate into proliferating chondrocytes and fibroblast-like cells in the perichondrium (**b**). **c** Chondrocytes form distinct subpopulations, which can be morphologically distinguished from distal to central into RP and CP chondrocytes. After cell cycle exit, chondrocytes differentiate into prehypertrophic, hypertrophic and terminal hypertrophic cells. Adjacent to the hypertrophic zone, cells in the perichondrium mineralize and form the periosteum. **d** Blood vessels invade the hypertrophic region and initiate bone formation in the center of the skeletal elements.

in columns (CP chondrocytes) towards the center [1–3]. In the center of the growing cartilage anlagen, chondrocytes exit the cell cycle and differentiate into prehypertrophic and hypertrophic chondrocytes (fig. 1c, 2a). These produce a mineralized extracellular cartilage matrix that serves as a template for the subsequent deposition of bone matrix. The increasing volume of the hypertrophic cells contributes significantly to the elongation of the skeletal elements.

The cartilage elements are surrounded by a layer of fibroblast-like cells, the perichondrium. At stages when chondrocytes become hypertrophic, cells in the perichondrium differentiate into osteoblasts forming the periost, which is highly vascularized. Blood vessels from the periost invade the calcified matrix of terminal hypertrophic chondrocytes, which undergo apoptosis. Together with the blood vessels osteoblasts and osteoclasts invade the skeletal elements to replace the mineralized cartilage by bone generating the primary spongiosa (fig. 1c, d) [4, 5]. In parallel, osteoblasts in the periost produce a calcified matrix forming the bone collar. The early bone collar and the primary trabecles are later remodeled to form the cortical bone and the bone marrow cavity, which provides a local environment for hematopoiesis.

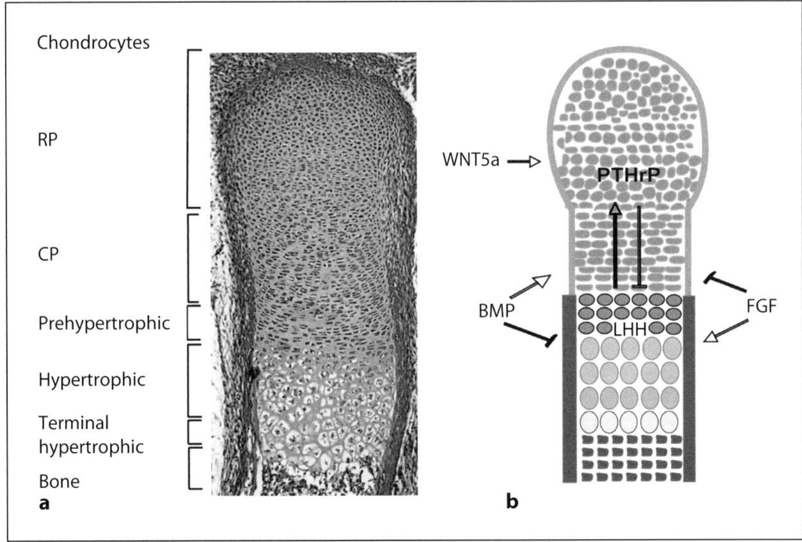

Fig. 2. In the embryonic growth plates, distinct chondrocyte populations can be morphologically distinguished. **a** Safranin-Weigert staining of a longitudinal section through an E16.5 mouse forelimb showing the characteristic morphology of the cartilage. **b** Schematic model of a longitudinal section through an embryonic growth plate showing the different chondrocyte subpopulations. Growth factors (BMP, FGF, IHH, PTHrP and WNT5a) can activate (arrows) or inhibit (bars) the formation of distinct chondrocyte populations.

During postnatal development, secondary ossification centers are formed within the zone of the RP chondrocytes (fig. 1d). Between the two ossification centers chondrocytes remain forming the postnatal growth plate. Many studies investigating postnatal growth plate differentiation strongly indicate that the mechanisms controlling the embryonic processes are maintained until adulthood [6].

Longitudinal growth of bones is dependent on the rate of chondrocyte proliferation, the size of the proliferating region and the expansion of the hypertrophic region. During embryonic and postnatal development, the balance between chondrocyte proliferation and differentiation has to be tightly controlled to ensure normal longitudinal bone growth and endochondral bone formation. Both, disturbed chondrocyte proliferation and hypertrophic differentiation, will lead to alterations in bone length and stability.

The sensitivity of the system is reflected by the large number of human chondrodysplasias and the multitude of transgenic mice that show skeletal defects [7]. During the last years, considerable progress has been made in analyzing the signals regulating endochondral ossification. However, the mechanisms by which these signals are translated into gene expression are less well understood. Here, we will summarize some of the relevant signaling pathways and concentrate on recent advances in deciphering the transcriptional network acting downstream of these pathways.

Regulation by Growth Factors

Indian Hedgehog Signaling

One of the key regulators of endochondral bone formation is the secreted growth factor IHH which is expressed in prehypertophic chondrocytes. IHH signals to the proliferating chondrocytes and to the periosteum. In proliferating chondrocytes, IHH signaling directly activates proliferation, especially in CP chondrocytes. In parallel, high IHH signals repress the expansion of the pool of RP chondrocytes, whereas low IHH levels favor its expansion. Furthermore, IHH induces the expression of PTHrP in RP chondrocytes. Activation of the PPR1, expressed in proliferating and prehypertrophic chondrocytes, by PTHrP prevents the onset of hypertrophic differentiation and, thus, the differentiation of IHH-expressing cells (fig. 2b) [8, 9]. By initiating this negative feedback system, IHH regulates the pool of proliferating cells in parallel to the proliferation rate.

Signaling of IHH is mediated by transcription factors of the GLI family, which consist of GLI1, GLI2 and GLI3. GLI1 activates IHH target genes, while GLI2 and GLI3 can function as activators or can be processed into a repressor form [10, 11]. This proteolytic processing is negatively regulated by IHH signaling leading to distinct levels of GLI activator and GLI repressor forms in different chondrocyte subpopulations.

Bone Morphogenetic Protein Signaling

BMPs were identified by their ability to induce ectopic endochondral ossification. Several members of the BMP family, which represents a subgroup of the transforming growth factor family of secreted proteins, and their receptors (BMPRs) are expressed in the cartilage anlagen [12]. BMP signaling is mediated by heteromeric complexes of type I (BM PR1a and BMPR1b) and type II (BMPR2) receptors. Activation of these receptor complexes leads to the phosphorylation of SMAD transcription factors SMAD1, SMAD5 and SMAD8. Phosphorylated SMAD proteins interact with the common mediator SMAD4 to activate transcription of target genes [13]. BMP signaling induces chondrocyte proliferation, whereas loss of both BMPR1a and 1b leads to hypoplastic cartilage anlagen, identifying BMPs as positive regulators of cell cycle progression [4, 14, 15].

Fibroblast Growth Factor Signaling

Like BMPs, FGFs are members of a large family of signaling proteins, which act at multiple steps of the differentiation process. FGF signaling leads to activation of the MAP pathway and phosphorylation of transcription factors of the STAT family, e.g. STAT1 [16, 17]. Constitutively activating mutations in the *FGFR3* lead to achondroplasia, one of the most common forms of human dwarfism. Mice mimicking the human mutation revealed that the constitutive activation of *FGFR3* inhibits chondrocyte proliferation and accelerates hypertrophic differentiation [18, 19]. In contrast, deletion of *FGFR3* or *FGF18* increases chondrocyte proliferation and expands the pool of hypertrophic cells [20]. Thus, FGF signaling seems to antagonize BMP function in many aspects (fig. 2b) [19, 21].

WNT Signaling

WNT signals have been shown to act on chondro-osseus progenitor cells of the early mesenchymal condensation. Activation of WNT signaling supports osteoblast differentiation and, simultaneously, prevents chondrocyte differentiation of mesenchymal cells [22, 23]. In differentiated chondrocytes, WNT signaling induces hypertrophic differentiation [24] and joint formation [25]. Canonical WNT signaling is mediated by the transcription factor β-catenin, while transcription factors acting downstream of noncanonical WNT signals have not been identified yet [22, 26].

Transcriptional Control of Cartilage Development

Mesenchymal Condensation

The differentiation of chondrocytes requires several cell fate decisions to establish the chondrogenic fate. The transcription factor SOX9, which belongs to the family of 'high-mobility group box' transcription factors, is one of the earliest markers of condensing chondrocytes. The expression of *SOX9* starts in chondroprogenitor cells and is maintained in proliferating chondrocytes. In humans, mutations in *SOX9* lead to campomelic dysplasia syndrome, which is characterized by severe malformations of the endochondral skeleton. In mice, heterozygous loss of *SOX9* results in hypoplastic skeletal elements, while homozygous deletion completely inhibits chondrogenesis [7]. Interestingly, in chimeric mice carrying *SOX9* mutant cells in a wild type background, *SOX9*-deficient cells are excluded from the cartilage condensations [27] indicating that SOX9 function is required to establish the chondrogenic lineage.

Another transcription factor regulating mesenchymal condensation is β-catenin, which acts downstream of WNT signals. Activation of WNT-signaling induces stabilization and nuclear translocation of β-catenin. Loss of β-catenin activity is required in mesenchymal cells to initiate chondrocyte differentiation. In these cells, stabilization of β-catenin represses *SOX9* expression preventing cartilage formation, whereas loss of β-catenin leads to defects in osteoblast formation [22]. The interaction between SOX9 and β-catenin thus balances the specification of chondrocytes versus osteoblasts (fig. 3a).

Patterning of the Cartilaginous Epiphysis

Once the chondrocyte cell type has been established, proliferating chondrocytes will differentiate into two cell types, RP chondrocytes and CP chondrocytes. The level of IHH-dependent PTHrP signaling has been shown to define the region of proliferating chondrocytes. However, closer inspection of mice expressing increased levels of *IHH* and, subsequently, PTHrP levels revealed a specific expansion of CP chondrocytes,

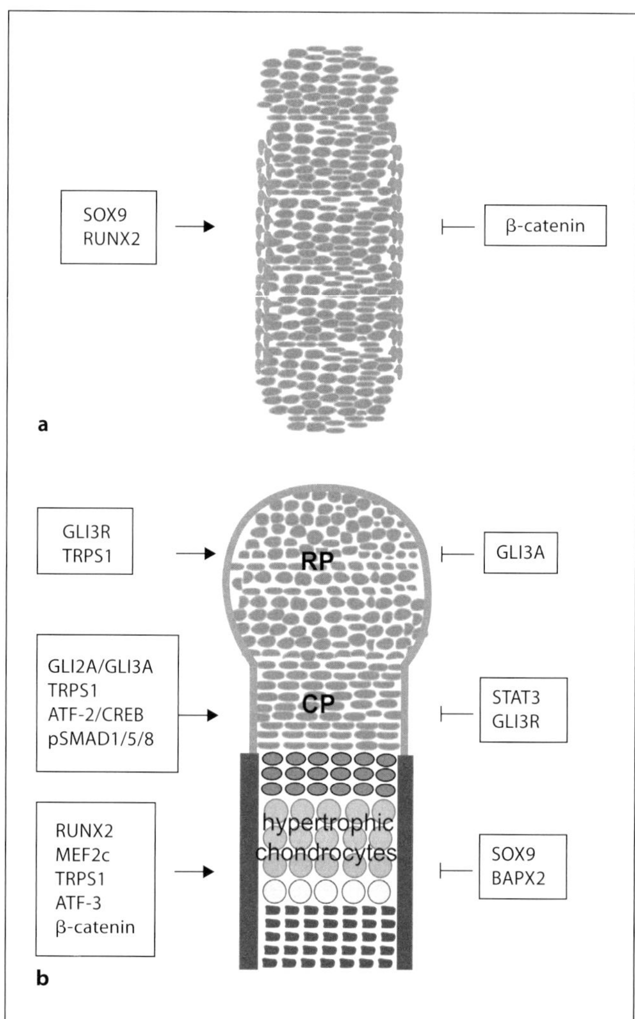

Fig. 3. Regulatory network of transcription factors which cooperate during mesenchymal condensation (**a**) and at subsequent steps of chondrocyte differentiation (RP, CP and hypertrophic chondrocytes; **b**).

whereas the region of RP chondrocytes is actually reduced [28, 29]. Mice deficient in *GLI3*, one of the transcription factors acting downstream of IHH signaling, show a decreased zone of RP chondrocytes. Similarly, IHH-dependent activation of GLI2 or GLI3 will not only increase *PTHrP* expression, but simultaneously reduce the zone of RP chondrocytes [28]. As GLI3 has been shown to act mainly as a repressor of IHH signaling, the balance between GLI3 repressor and GLI2/GLI3 activator seems to determine the pool of RP versus CP chondrocytes [28, 30].

Besides GLI3, the GATA-type transcription factor TRPS1 plays an important role in proliferating chondrocytes. Different studies demonstrated that TRPS1 inhibits chondrocyte proliferation [31–33]. Nevertheless, the zone of CP chondrocytes is not shortened, but slightly increased. Accordingly, *PTHrP* expression is not reduced, supporting the hypothesis that PTHrP signaling specifically regulates the region of CP cells independent of the proliferation rate. The region of RP cells is similarly decreased in *TRPS1* and *GLI3* mutants identifying TRPS1 as a second transcription factor regulating the pool of RP chondrocytes [31]. Interestingly, TRPS1 has been shown to specifically interact with the activator form of GLI3. Whether this interaction leads to an inactivation of the GLI3 activator, thereby shifting the balance towards the GLI3 repressor, will be a challenging question for future studies.

In addition to these transcription factors, noncanonical WNT signaling induced by WNT5a and WNT5b, seems to regulate the region of proliferating chondrocytes (fig. 2b). In *WNT5a*-deficient mice, the proliferation rate and region of RP chondrocytes is reduced, indicating that WNT5a regulates the pool of RP chondrocytes independent of IHH/PTHrP signaling [26].

Chondrocyte Proliferation

The rate of chondrocyte proliferation is regulated by cyclins, forming complexes with CDKs. These complexes phosphorylate pRB, p107 and p130, members of the pocket protein family, which bind to E2F transcription factors as unphosphorylated proteins. Upon phosphorylation, E2F is released and translocates to the nucleus, where it activates the expression of cell cycle-promoting target genes. Complex formation of cyclins and CDKs is repressed by cyclin-dependent kinase inhibitors (CDKIs), including p21, p27 and p57 proteins [34]. Various loss and gain of function studies of cell cycle regulators have identified growth and differentiation defects in transgenic mice [35–37]. Cyclin D1-deficient mice develop dwarfism and a reduced zone of proliferating chondrocytes [38]. Another example is the overexpression of the negative cell cycle regulator p21, which leads to premature induction of chondrocyte differentiation in cell culture experiments [39].

IHH and PTHrP have been shown to regulate cell cycle progression by activation of cyclins. *IHH*-overexpressing mice show an increased proliferation rate and cyclin D1 expression, while both are severely decreased in *IHH*-deficient mutants [1]. Accordingly, the analysis of mouse mutants showed that GLI2 acts as an activator of chondrocyte proliferation, while loss of *GLI3* has negligible effects on chondrocyte proliferation [40]. Nevertheless, loss of *GLI3* in *IHH*-deficient mice rescues the reduced proliferation rate of *IHH* mutants [28, 41]. Together, these data indicate that the balance between GLI repressor and activator forms is critical to regulate chondrocyte proliferation downstream of IHH signaling. Supporting evidence comes from cell culture experiments demonstrating that the GLI3 repressor can directly bind to the cyclin D1 promoter in kidney cells [42]. However, a direct regulation of cyclin D1 in chondrocytes in vivo has not been demonstrated yet.

In parallel to regulating the region of CP chondrocytes, PTHrP can directly activate the chondrocyte proliferation rate. The family of ATF/ CREB induces chondrocyte proliferation downstream of PTHrP signaling [43, 44]. Supporting these data, *ATF-2-* and *CREB*-deficient mice develop dwarfism, characterized by shortened growth plates and kyphosis [45, 46]. In vitro PTHrP signaling induces phosphorylation of CREB by protein kinase A. Phosphorylated CREB activates cyclin D1 and E2F and, thus, cell cycle progression of chondrocytes [47].

Interestingly, TRPS1, which interacts with GLI3 in regulating the pool of RP chondrocytes, seems to act in parallel to GLI2/GLI3 to regulate the proliferation rate. In *TRPS1*-deficient mice, the reduced chondrocyte proliferation cannot be rescued by loss of *GLI3*, but increased IHH signaling can activate chondrocyte proliferation in *TRPS1* mutants [31]. It is thus likely that TRPS1- and IHH-dependent GLI transcription factors act at different steps of cell cycle progression.

In parallel to IHH and PTHrP, BMP signaling can activate chondrocyte proliferation by phosphorylation and activation of SMAD transcription factors. [13]. Deletion of individual *SMADS* results in viable and fertile mice [48], whereas *SMAD1, SMAD5* and *SMAD8* compound mutants develop severe cartilage hypoplasia due to reduced chondrocyte proliferation and an accelerated onset of hypertrophic differentiation. While a direct regulation of hypertrophic differentiation markers by BMP-responsive SMADs has been reported [48], the mechanisms by which SMAD proteins regulate proliferation on a transcriptional level have not been analyzed in detail.

The induction of chondrocyte proliferation by BMP signaling can be antagonized by FGFs. FGFs negatively regulate chondrocyte proliferation by phosphorylation of the transcription factor STAT1 [16, 17] resulting in increased expression of the pocket proteins p107 and p130 and the cell cycle inhibitor p21 [49, 50] and consequently an arrest in cell cycle progression. BMP signaling interferes with FGF-mediated repression of proliferation by a negative regulation of STAT1 and MAP kinase signaling [21].

Similar to FGF, WNT5a signaling upregulates the cell cycle inhibitor p130. Additionally, WNT5a suppresses cyclin D1 expression [26] which might be a mechanism by which WNT5a opposes IHH-induced activation of chondrocyte proliferation.

Hypertrophic Differentiation

Hypertrophic differentiation of chondrocytes requires cell cycle exit, the loss of differentiation inhibiting signals and activation of inducing factors. The IHH/PTHrP system acts in proliferating chondrocytes to prevent hypertrophic differentiation. Clonal loss of PPR1 in single cells will induce hypertrophic differentiation in a wild type environment, indicating that PTHrP signals act cell autonomously to block hypertrophic differentiation [51]. A main inducer of hypertrophic differentiation is the transcription factor RUNX2, which is expressed in prehypertrophic and hypertrophic chondrocytes. Homozygous deletion of *RUNX2* in mice results in delayed chondrocyte maturation. This delay is enhanced if *RUNX3 i*s deleted in addition [52]. No hypertrophic cells can be detected in *RUNX2;RUNX3* double mutants. In contrast, overexpression of *RUNX2* is sufficient to initiate hypertrophic differentiation [53]. A downstream target of RUNX2 is the MEF2c, which, like RUNX2, is essential for hypertrophic chondrocyte formation [54].

Interestingly, the increased expression of RUNX2 in prehypertrophic chondrocytes is coupled to cell cycle progression. In proliferating chondrocytes, the cyclin D1/CDK4 complexes mediate the degradation of RUNX2 protein, restricting hypertrophic differentiation to postproliferative cells only [55]. Cell cycle exit is triggered by the transcription factor ATF-3, which represses cyclin D1 and cyclin A [56], thereby allowing increased RUNX2 expression. In addition, SOX9, which supports the proliferating cell type and negatively regulates RUNX2 expression in proliferating cells, has to be inactivated to induce hypertrophy. While IHH has been reported to be induced by RUNX2 in hypertrophic chondrocytes [52], PTHrP expression is regulated by SOX9 linking the hypertrophy-inhibiting [57] IHH/PTHrP system to these transcriptional regulators.

References

1 Long F, Zhang XM, Karp S, Yang Y, McMahon AP: Genetic manipulation of hedgehog signaling in the endochondral skeleton reveals a direct role in the regulation of chondrocyte proliferation. Development 2001;128:5099–5108.

2 Kobayashi T, Chung UI, Schipani E, Starbuck M, Karsenty G, Katagiri T, Goad DL, Lanske B, Kronenberg HM: PTHrP and Indian hedgehog control differentiation of growth plate chondrocytes at multiple steps. Development 2002;129:2977–2986.

3 MacLean HE, Kronenberg HM: Localization of Indian hedgehog and PTH/PTHrP receptor expression in relation to chondrocyte proliferation during mouse bone development. Dev Growth Differ 2005; 47:59–63.

4 Hall BK, Miyake T: Divide, accumulate, differentiate: cell condensation in skeletal development revisited. Int J Dev Biol 1995;39:881–893.

5 Hall BK, Miyake T: All for one and one for all: condensations and the initiation of skeletal development. Bioessays 2000;22:138–147.

6 Cohen MM Jr: The new bone biology: pathologic, molecular, and clinical correlates. Am J Med Genet A 2006;140:2646–2706.

7 Goldring MB, Tsuchimochi K, Ijiri K: The control of chondrogenesis. J Cell Biochem 2006;97:33–44.

8 Vortkamp A, Lee K, Lanske B, Segre GV, Kronenberg HM, Tabin CJ: Regulation of rate of cartilage differentiation by Indian hedgehog and PTH-related protein. Science 1996;273:613–622.

9 St-Jacques B, Hammerschmidt M, McMahon AP: Indian hedgehog signaling regulates proliferation and differentiation of chondrocytes and is essential for bone formation. Genes Dev 1999;13:2072–2086.

10 Pan Y, Wang C, Wang B: Phosphorylation of Gli2 by protein kinase A is required for Gli2 processing and degradation and the Sonic Hedgehog-regulated mouse development. Dev Biol 2009;326:177–189.

11 Pan Y, Wang B: A novel protein-processing domain in Gli2 and Gli3 differentially blocks complete protein degradation by the proteasome. J Biol Chem 2007;282:10846–10852.

12 Minina E, Schneider S, Rosowski M, Lauster R, Vortkamp A: Expression of Fgf and Tgfbeta signaling related genes during embryonic endochondral ossification. Gene Expr Patterns 2005;6:102–109.

13 Goumans MJ, Mummery C: Functional analysis of the TGFbeta receptor/Smad pathway through gene ablation in mice. Int J Dev Biol 2000;44:253–265.

14 Yoon BS, Lyons KM: Multiple functions of BMPs in chondrogenesis. J Cell Biochem 2004;93:93–103.

15 Yoon BS, Ovchinnikov DA, Yoshii I, Mishina Y, Behringer RR, Lyons KM: Bmpr1a and Bmpr1b have overlapping functions and are essential for chondrogenesis in vivo. Proc Natl Acad Sci U S A 2005;102:5062–5067.

16 Sahni M, Raz R, Coffin JD, Levy D, Basilico C: STAT1 mediates the increased apoptosis and reduced chondrocyte proliferation in mice overexpressing FGF2. Development 2001;128:2119–2129.

17 Murakami S, Balmes G, McKinney S, Zhang Z, Givol D, de Crombrugghe B: Constitutive activation of MEK1 in chondrocytes causes Stat1-independent achondroplasia-like dwarfism and rescues the Fgfr3-deficient mouse phenotype. Genes Dev 2004; 18:290–305.

18 Yamaguchi TP, Rossant J: Fibroblast growth factors in mammalian development. Curr Opin Genet Dev 1995;5:485–491.

19 Minina E, Kreschel C, Naski MC, Ornitz DM, Vortkamp A: Interaction of FGF, Ihh/Pthlh, and BMP signaling integrates chondrocyte proliferation and hypertrophic differentiation. Dev Cell 2002;3: 439–449.

20 Liu Z, Lavine KJ, Hung IH, Ornitz DM: FGF18 is required for early chondrocyte proliferation, hypertrophy and vascular invasion of the growth plate. Dev Biol 2007;302:80–91.

21 Yoon BS, Pogue R, Ovchinnikov DA, Yoshii I, Mishina Y, Behringer RR, Lyons KM: BMPs regulate multiple aspects of growth-plate chondrogenesis through opposing actions on FGF pathways. Development 2006;133:4667–4678.

22 Hill TP, Später D, Taketo MM, Birchmeier W, Hartmann C: Canonical Wnt/beta-catenin signaling prevents osteoblasts from differentiating into chondrocytes. Dev Cell 2005;8:727–738.

23 Reinhold MI, Kapadia RM, Liao Z, Naski MC: The Wnt-inducible transcription factor Twist1 inhibits chondrogenesis. J Biol Chem 2006;281:1381–1388.

24 Guo X, Mak KK, Taketo MM, Yang Y: The Wnt/beta-catenin pathway interacts differentially with PTHrP signaling to control chondrocyte hypertrophy and final maturation. PLoS One 2009;4:e6067.

25 Hartmann C: Skeletal development – Wnts are in control. Mol Cells 2007;24:177–184.

26 Yang Y, Topol L, Lee H, Wu J: Wnt5a and Wnt5b exhibit distinct activities in coordinating chondrocyte proliferation and differentiation. Development 2003;130:1003–1015.

27 Bi W, Deng JM, Zhang Z, Behringer RR, de Crombrugghe B: Sox9 is required for cartilage formation. Nat Genet 1999;22:85–89.

28 Koziel L, Wuelling M, Schneider S, Vortkamp A: Gli3 acts as a repressor downstream of Ihh in regulating two distinct steps of chondrocyte differentiation. Development 2005;132:5249–5260.

29 Kobayashi T, Soegiarto DW, Yang Y, Lanske B, Schipani E, McMahon AP, Kronenberg HM: Indian hedgehog stimulates periarticular chondrocyte differentiation to regulate growth plate length independently of PTHrP. J Clin Invest 2005;115: 1734–1742.

30 Kesper DA, Didt-Koziel L, Vortkamp A: Gli2 activator function in preosteoblasts is sufficient to mediate Ihh-dependent osteoblast differentiation, whereas the repressor function of Gli2 is dispensable for endochondral ossification. Dev Dyn 2010; 239:1818–1826.

31 Wuelling M, Kaiser FJ, Buelens LA, Braunholz D, Shivdasani RA, Depping R, Vortkamp A: Trps1, a regulator of chondrocyte proliferation and differentiation, interacts with the activator form of Gli3. Dev Biol 2009;328:40–53.

32 Suemoto H, Muragaki Y, Nishioka K, Sato M, Ooshima A, Itoh S, Hatamura I, Ozaki M, Braun A, Gustafsson E, Fässler R: Trps1 regulates proliferation and apoptosis of chondrocytes through Stat3 signaling. Dev Biol 2007;312:572–581.

33 Napierala D, Sam K, Morello R, Zheng Q, Munivez E, Shivdasani RA, Lee B: Uncoupling of chondrocyte differentiation and perichondrial mineralization underlies the skeletal dysplasia in tricho-rhino-phalangeal syndrome. Hum Mol Genet 2008;17: 2244–2254.

34 LuValle P, Beier F: Cell cycle control in growth plate chondrocytes. Front Biosci 2000;5:D493–D503.

35 Sherr CJ, Roberts JM: Living with or without cyclins and cyclin-dependent kinases. Genes Dev 2004;18: 2699–2711.

36 Rossi F, MacLean HE, Yuan W, Francis RO, Semenova E, Lin CS, Kronenberg HM, Cobrinik D: p107 and p130 coordinately regulate proliferation, Cbfa1 expression, and hypertrophic differentiation during endochondral bone development. Dev Biol 2002;247:271–285.

37 Scheijen B, Bronk M, van der Meer T, Bernards R: Constitutive E2F1 overexpression delays endochondral bone formation by inhibiting chondrocyte differentiation. Mol Cell Biol 2003;23:3656–3668.

38 Beier F, Ali Z, Mok D, Taylor AC, Leask T, Albanese C, Pestell RG, LuValle P: TGFbeta and PTHrP control chondrocyte proliferation by activating cyclin D1 expression. Mol Biol Cell 2001;12:3852–3863.

39 Nakajima M, Negishi Y, Tanaka H, Kawashima K: p21(Cip-1/SDI-1/WAF-1) expression via the mitogen-activated protein kinase signaling pathway in insulin-induced chondrogenic differentiation of ATDC5 cells. Biochem Biophys Res Commun 2004; 320:1069–1075.

40 Mau E, Whetstone H, Yu C, Hopyan S, Wunder JS, Alman BA: PTHrP regulates growth plate chondrocyte differentiation and proliferation in a Gli3 dependent manner utilizing hedgehog ligand dependent and independent mechanisms. Dev Biol 2007;305:28–39.

41 Hilton MJ, Tu X, Cook J, Hu H, Long F: Ihh controls cartilage development by antagonizing Gli3, but requires additional effectors to regulate osteoblast and vascular development. Development 2005;132:4339–4351.
42 Hu MC, Mo R, Bhella S, Wilson CW, Chuang PT, Hui CC, Rosenblum ND: GLI3-dependent transcriptional repression of Gli1, Gli2 and kidney patterning genes disrupts renal morphogenesis. Development 2006;133:569–578.
43 Provot S, Nachtrab G, Paruch J, Chen AP, Silva A, Kronenberg HM: A-raf and B-raf are dispensable for normal endochondral bone development, and parathyroid hormone-related peptide suppresses extracellular signal-regulated kinase activation in hypertrophic chondrocytes. Mol Cell Biol 2008;28:344–357.
44 Long F, Schipani E, Asahara H, Kronenberg H, Montminy M: The CREB family of activators is required for endochondral bone development. Development 2001;128:541–550.
45 Provot S, Schipani E: Molecular mechanisms of endochondral bone development. Biochem Biophys Res Commun 2005;328:658–665.
46 Reimold AM, Grusby MJ, Kosaras B, Fries JW, Mori R, Maniwa S, Clauss IM, Collins T, Sidman RL, Glimcher MJ, Glimcher LH: Chondrodysplasia and neurological abnormalities in ATF-2-deficient mice. Nature 1996;379:262–265.
47 Beier F, LuValle P: The cyclin D1 and cyclin A genes are targets of activated PTH/PTHrP receptors in Jansen's metaphyseal chondrodysplasia. Mol Endocrinol 2002;16:2163–2173.
48 Retting KN, Song B, Yoon BS, Lyons KM: BMP canonical Smad signaling through Smad1 and Smad5 is required for endochondral bone formation. Development 2009;136:1093–1104.
49 Dailey L, Laplantine E, Priore R, Basilico C: A network of transcriptional and signaling events is activated by FGF to induce chondrocyte growth arrest and differentiation. J Cell Biol 2003;161:1053–1066.
50 Dailey L, Ambrosetti D, Mansukhani A, Basilico C: Mechanisms underlying differential responses to FGF signaling. Cytokine Growth Factor Rev 2005;16:233–247.
51 Chung UI, Lanske B, Lee K, Li E, Kronenberg H: The parathyroid hormone/parathyroid hormone-related peptide receptor coordinates endochondral bone development by directly controlling chondrocyte differentiation. Proc Natl Acad Sci U S A 1998;95:13030–13035.
52 Yoshida CA, Yamamoto H, Fujita T, Furuichi T, Ito K, Inoue K, Yamana K, Zanma A, Takada K, Ito Y, Komori T: Runx2 and Runx3 are essential for chondrocyte maturation, and Runx2 regulates limb growth through induction of Indian hedgehog. Genes Dev 2004;18:952–963.
53 Komori T: Regulation of skeletal development by the Runx family of transcription factors. J Cell Biochem 2005;95:445–453.
54 Arnold MA, Kim Y, Czubryt MP, Phan D, McAnally J, Qi X, Shelton JM, Richardson JA, Bassel-Duby R, Olson EN: MEF2C transcription factor controls chondrocyte hypertrophy and bone development. Dev Cell 2007;12:377–389.
55 Zhang S, Xiao Z, Luo J, He N, Mahlios J, Quarles LD: Dose-dependent effects of Runx2 on bone development. J Bone Miner Res 2009;24:1889–1904.
56 James CG, Appleton CT, Ulici V, Underhill TM, Beier F: Microarray analyses of gene expression during chondrocyte differentiation identifies novel regulators of hypertrophy. Mol Biol Cell 2005;16:5316–33.
57 Amano K, Hata K, Sugita A, Takigawa Y, Ono K, Wakabayashi M, Kogo M, Nishimura R, Yoneda T: Sox9 family members negatively regulate maturation and calcification of chondrocytes through up-regulation of parathyroid hormone-related protein. Mol Biol Cell 2009;20:4541–4551.

Prof. Dr. Andrea Vortkamp
Center for Medical Biotechnology, Department of Developmental Biology, University Duisburg-Essen
DE–45117 Essen (Germany)
Tel. +49 201 183 4298, Fax +49 201 183 3852, E-Mail andrea.vortkamp@uni-due.de

Camacho-Hübner C, Nilsson O, Sävendahl L (eds): Cartilage and Bone Development and Its Disorders.
Endocr Dev. Basel, Karger, 2011, vol 21, pp 12–22

Local Regulation of Growth Plate Cartilage

Stephan-Stanislaw Späth · Anenisia C. Andrade · Michael Chau · Ola Nilsson

Center for Molecular Medicine and Pediatric Endocrinology Unit, Q2:08, Department of Women's and Children's Health, Karolinska Institutet and University Hospital, Stockholm, Sweden

Abstract

Elongation of bones primarily occurs by endochondral ossification at the growth plate. In the growth plate, stem-like cells in the resting zone differentiate into rapidly dividing chondrocytes in the proliferative zone and then terminally differentiate into nondividing chondrocytes of the hypertrophic zone. The hypertrophic zone is then invaded by blood vessels and bone cell precursors, which remodel the newly formed cartilage into bone. The net effect is that new bone tissue is progressively generated at the bottom of the growth plate, resulting in bone elongation. The process of longitudinal bone growth is governed by a complex network of paracrine signals that maintain the unique structure and cellular kinetics of the growth plate. Recent progress in the understanding of important paracrine signals that regulate growth plate cartilage will be reviewed in this chapter.

Longitudinal bone growth occurs at the growth plate by endochondral bone formation in which cartilage is first formed and then remodeled into bone. The growth plate contains one cell type, the chondrocyte, at different stages of differentiation that are spatially separated, forming a structure with three histologically distinct cell layers: resting, proliferative and hypertrophic zones. The resting zone chondrocytes replicate at a slow rate [1] and act as stem-like cells that replenish the pool of proliferative chondrocytes [2]. Proliferative zone chondrocytes, on the other hand, replicate at a high rate [1], and the newly generated daughter cells line up along the long axis of the bone. As a result, chondrocyte clones are arranged in columns parallel to this axis, a process which is critical to bone elongation [2].

The hypertrophic zone contains terminally differentiated chondrocytes which calcify their surrounding ECM and attract invading bone and endothelial cells, a crucial step in endochondral bone formation.

At a certain point, the cells stop dividing and terminally differentiate into hypertrophic chondrocytes [1]. During the hypertrophic process, chondrocytes increase their height about 6- to 10-fold, and hence this hypertrophic differentiation significantly contributes to longitudinal bone growth [3]. In addition, hypertrophic chondrocytes prepare the cartilage for remodeling into bone by calcifying the surrounding ECM and by producing enzymes that help digest the collagenous components of the matrix [3]. The hypertrophic chondrocytes also produce several factors, including VEGF that attracts invading bone cells and blood vessels [4]. Hypertrophic chondrocytes undergo apoptosis shortly before the blood vessels invade the chondrocyte lacuna [5].

The unique cellular architecture and kinetics of the growth plate requires both patterning and differentiating factors that act together to regulate the process of growth plate chondrogenesis. The understanding of these regulatory signals has increased substantially over the past few years. The role of PTHrP, IHH, BMPs, FGFs, and WNT signaling in growth plate chondrogenesis will be discussed below. The role of IHH and PTHrP has been evaluated by careful studies using genetically modified animals and fetal organ culture systems. The importance of the BMP, FGF and WNT signaling in endochondral bone formation is clear, but the large number of ligands and their receptors in these systems has so far not permitted a straightforward approach to elucidate the exact role of the individual factors involved.

Parathyroid Hormone-Related Protein

PTHrP was originally discovered in association with humoral hypercalcemia of malignancy. The protein mimics the actions of PTH by virtue of having N-terminal homology (amino acids 1–34) and thus signals via the same receptor, PTH1R [6]. In the growth plate, PTHrP, signaling through PTH1R, inhibits hypertrophic differentiation of proliferative chondrocytes, thereby maintaining them in a proliferative mode. Mice in which either the PTHrP or the PTH1R gene was ablated exhibit similar abnormalities in the growth plate. Both have short limbs and thin proliferative zones with hypertrophic chondrocytes close to the ends of the bones, suggesting accelerated chondrocyte maturation [7, 8]. Conversely, overexpression of PTHrP results in short limbs due to a delay in chondrocyte maturation [9]. In chimeric mice containing wild-type and PTH1R–/– chondrocytes, the PTH1R–/– proliferative chondrocytes underwent hypertrophic differentiation while still located in the proliferative zone, confirming the important regulatory role of PTH1R signaling in chondrocyte differentiation in vivo [10].

The PTH1R appears to play a similar role in human skeletal development, since mutations in the PTHrP receptor cause at least two different conditions with altered chondrocyte maturation. Null mutations of the PTH1R, such as in Blomstrand lethal osteochondrodysplasia, are associated with accelerated maturation and ossification of the developing skeleton [11, 12], which resemble the skeletal phenotype of PTH1R–/– mice. Jansen's metaphyseal chondrodysplasia, an autosomal dominant disorder that is characterized by short limb dwarfism, hypercalcemia, and hypophosphatemia, is caused by activating mutations of PTH1R [13].

Indian Hedgehog

IHH belongs to the three-member Hedgehog family of secreted morphogens that is essential for multiple developmental processes [14]. Genetic targeting of IHH, PTHrP, and PTH1R has revealed a mechanism by which the balance between proliferation and differentiation is controlled, at least during fetal development [15]. IHH is predominantly secreted by early hypertrophic chondrocytes and PTHrP by periarticular chondrocytes, whereas the PTH1R is expressed by proliferative and hypertrophic chondrocytes [16, 17]. IHH produced by newly formed hypertrophic chondrocytes signals to periarticular epiphyseal chondrocytes, inducing them to synthesize PTHrP. PTHrP then acts on the PTHR1 on proliferative chondrocytes to inhibit their differentiation into hypertrophic chondrocytes, thus forming a feedback loop that stabilizes the rate of chondrocyte differentiation and consequently the height of the proliferative columns [15, 16, 18, 19]. At around the time of birth, PTHrP expression moves into the resting zones and the feedback loop may thus be maintained when the secondary ossification center is formed [20]. Independent of PTHrP signaling, IHH also stimulates chondrocyte proliferation and promotes differentiation of resting chondrocytes [16, 21]. In addition, IHH signaling couples chondrogenesis to osteogenesis by inducing bone collar formation in the perichondrium adjacent to the IHH expressing chondrocytes, presumably by a direct effect on osteoblast differentiation [10, 16].

Recent reports have suggested an essential role for IHH in normal human skeletal development. Mutations in the IHH gene are linked to at least two inherited skeletal development disorders: ACFD an autosomal recessive disorder characterized by short limbed dwarfism, and conical epiphyses in the hands and hips [22] and BDA1, an autosomal dominant disorder, characterized by shortened or absent middle phalanges in the digits. Both ACFD and BDA1 are associated with missense mutations in the region of the IHH gene encoding the amino-terminal signaling domain, which impair the interaction of IHH with its receptor, patched1 (Ptch1) [23].

Fibroblast Growth Factors

FGFs are a large family of structurally related proteins that play important roles in development, homeostasis, wound healing, tissue repair as well as serum phosphate levels and vitamin D metabolism [24]. The first discoveries of FGF can be traced back to the 1930s, when bovine brain extracts have been shown to promote proliferation of

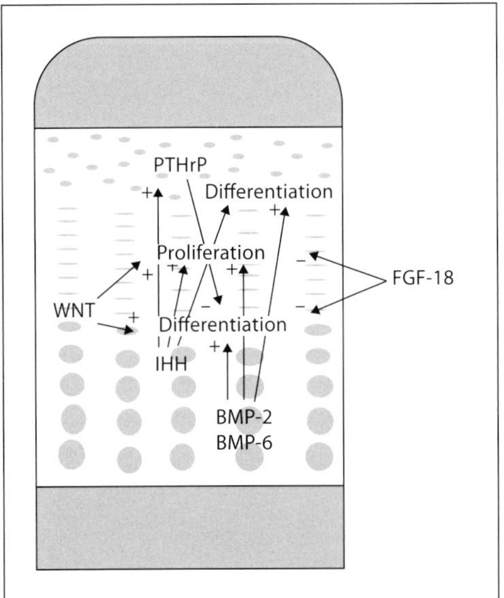

Fig. 1. Paracrine regulation of the growth plate. PTHrP secreted in the resting zone inhibits differentiation of proliferative chondrocytes. PTHrP production is in turn stimulated by IHH secreted by early hypertrophic chondrocytes. IHH and PTHrP form a feedback loop that acts to delay hypertrophic differentiation and consequently increases the height of the proliferative columns. IHH also stimulate chondrocyte differentiation of resting zone chondrocytes and proliferation of proliferative chondrocytes directly. FGF, exemplified by FGF-18 that is expressed in the perichondrium, inhibits both proliferation and differentiation of growth plate chondrocytes. BMPs produced by hypertrophic chondrocytes, stimulate differentiation of resting and proliferative chondrocytes and proliferation of proliferative chondrocytes. WNTs, expressed primarily by proliferative and early hypertrophic chondrocytes, promote proliferation and hypertrophic differentiation through the canonical β-catenin pathway. + = Stimulatory effect; – = inhibitory effect.

fibroblast cell lines in vitro [25]. Since then, 22 secreted members have been identified that can be classified into three subfamilies: (1) canonical FGFs (FGF1–10, 16–18, 20 and 22); (2) hormone-like FGFs (FGF15/19, 21, 23), and (3) intracellular FGFs (FGF11–14) [26]. Canonical FGFs bind to and activate high-affinity FGFRs, of which there are four identified members, FGFR1–4, predominantly in a paracrine fashion. All known FGFRs are transmembrane proteins, marked by an extracellular ligand-binding domain with three immunoglobulin-like domains with heparin/or heparan sulphate proteoglycan-binding capacity and an intracellular domain with tyrosine kinase activity [24, 25]. Numerous signaling pathways have been implicated following FGFR activation and include the signal transducer and activation of transcription, MAP, phospholipase Cγ, phosphoinositide 3 kinase, protein kinase C and the AKT pathways. What pathway and how strong the signaling effect will be, is highly dependent on a particular receptor (e.g. phosphorylation state and receptor stability), cellular content, cell development and metabolic state, as well as the input of signals from other signaling pathways (e.g. BMPs, WNTs and TGF-β; described later). It should be also mentioned that while heparin and/or heparan sulfate proteoglycans appear to bind with high affinity to canonical FGFs, hormone-like FGFs exhibit only weak affinities for heparin sites and likely act on target cells elsewhere in the body in an endocrine manner [24]. In addition, this weak binding requires the recruitment of other cell surface coreceptors (e.g. β-Klotho) that are synthesized by the corresponding target cells. Intracellular FGFs appear to act in an FGFR-independent manner and hence will not be discussed here.

The expression of FGFs as well as FGFRs and its role in limb development has been demonstrated in various species, including human. FGFR2 expression starts in condensing mesenchymal stem cells, in the central core of the developing limb, while FGFR1 tends to locate in the periphery of the condensing center. During further skeletal development, FGFR1 and FGFR2 expressions are shifted to the perichondrium and periosteum, and FGFR1 remains to be expressed in hypertrophic chondrocytes in the epiphyseal growth plate. In contrast, FGFR3 expression is first detectable during signs of chondrogenesis and remains expressed in proliferating chondrocytes [27]. During postnatal life, the isoform c of FGFR1, 2 and 3 predominates in the growth plate. FGFR1 and 3 are considered as negative regulators, whereas FGFR2 and 4 are putative positive regulators of growth plate chondrogenesis. FGFR2 and 4 are expressed in the RZ, FGFR3 and 4 in the PZ, and FGFR1 and 3 are expressed in HZ [28]. In general, FGF expression is low in growth plate chondrocytes, whereas FGF1, 2, 6, 7, 9, and 18 are expressed at high levels in the perichondrium [29–32].

Genetic targeting of the majority of FGFs has been attempted in animal models resulting in phenotypes ranging from no detectable abnormality to lethality. Excluding all lethal phenotypes at the embryonic stages, skeletal abnormalities in the murine offspring have been detected for FGF2, FGF18 and FGF23 knockouts. Since the discovery that achondroplasia, the most common form of human dwarfism, is caused by an activating point mutation in the transmembrane domain of FGFR3, a number of other skeletal dysplasias has been attributed to mutations in FGFR1, 2, and 3.

Similar to humans, murine models expressing activating mutations of the FGRFR-3 gene exhibit the syndrome, including short limb dwarfism due to decreased chondrocyte proliferation [33]. Conversely, FGFR-3 null mice show increased longitudinal bone growth, increased chondrocyte proliferation and taller proliferative columns in the growth plate [34]. In addition, ablation of FGFR3 results in an increase in IHH expression, while FGFR3 activation results in downregulation of IHH in murine animal models.

Mice with targeted disruption of FGF-18, like FGFR3-deficient mice, exhibit expanded proliferative and hypertrophic zones. In addition, *FGF18*-deficient mice show delayed ossification. This delay is not observed in FGFR3-deficient mice and may reflect a lack of FGFR1 activation in hypertrophic chondrocytes. These findings suggest that FGF-18 is the natural ligand for FGFR3 in the growth plate cartilage responsible for the inhibition of proliferative activity [35]. With age, as growth decelerates, FGFR2 and 4 are downregulated, and FGF1, 7, 18 and 22 are upregulated in the proliferative zone. These age-dependent changes may contribute to the decline in longitudinal bone growth that occurs with age [28].

Bone Morphogenetic Protein

BMPs were first discovered as the component of demineralized bone matrix that is able to induce new bone formation in intramuscular sites [36]. These proteins were later found to exhibit diverse roles during early embryogenesis, organogenesis and dorsal-ventral patterning by their ability to regulate cell proliferation, differentiation, apoptosis, and cell fate [20, 37]. BMPs are multifunctional growth factors that belong to the TGF-β superfamily, the largest group of growth factors in humans. Up to date, at least 20 BMPs are known and well characterized, with only BMPs 2–7 belonging to this family. The binding of BMPs to type I cell membrane receptors results in three signals, known as type IA, IB and ALK-2, that eventually lead to the activation of the canonical SMAD pathway as well as other signaling pathways [38].

BMP signaling governs numerous aspects of limb formation and outgrowth, including mesenchymal condensation, chondrocyte differentiation and apoptosis [39, 40]. To be able to play these diverse roles during development, BMP signaling has to be locally restricted by distinct expression of BMP antagonists. Genetic targeting in mice has revealed that loss of BMP antagonism by gremlin results in defective patterning and outgrowth of limbs [41] and that the BMP antagonist noggin is required for proper allocation of limb mesenchyme to the cartilage compartment and for specification of joints [36]. Similarly, in humans, heterozygous mutations of noggin result in a variety of skeletal abnormalities, including synostosis, symphalangism and abnormal joint formation. In the growth plate, BMP signaling promotes chondrocyte proliferation as well as differentiation of RZ to PZ chondrocytes and PZ to HZ chondrocytes [42, 43]. In the growth plate, BMP2 and 6 are highly expressed in hypertrophic chondrocytes, whereas BMP7 is primarily expressed in PZ chondrocytes. In contrast, gremlin, chordin and BMP3, all inhibiting factors of BMP-induced bone formation, are expressed at high levels in the RZ [44]. These expression profiles suggest a BMP signaling gradient in the growth plate that may contribute to maintain the spatial regulation of proliferation and differentiation in growth plate cartilage.

BMP signaling pathway and its mediators may interact directly or indirectly with other signaling pathways in the growth plate, in particular with the IHH/PTHrP and FGF pathways. The interaction of BMPs with the IHH/PTHrP pathway promotes IHH expression, which in turn appears to maintain BMP levels, pointing towards the existence of a positive feedback loop [45]. However, this should be treated with caution as neither pathway completely mediates the other's function and proceeds more in a synergistic way. BMPs and FGFs may also act as antagonists in chondrocyte regulation. While recombinant BMP treatment rescues the FGF-treated phenotype of the growth plates, the FGF treatment results in the opposite effect, by neutralizing the effect of BMPs [46]. The precise mechanism governing this antagonism is not well understood.

WNT Signaling

The importance of WNT signaling in skeletal development has been evaluated by several in vivo and in vitro studies [47]. WNTs, consisting of at least 19 members, comprise a complex family of secreted cysteine-rich glycoproteins that interact with several receptors, including frizzled (Fzd) and co-receptors Lrp5 and Lrp6. They are regulated by antagonists, e.g. secreted frizzled-related proteins (Sfrps), to finally activate different signaling pathways, including the calcium-releasing, JNK/planner cell polarity and the canonical WNT/β-catenin pathways. In the canonical WNT/β-catenin pathway, WNT signals stabilize β-catenin followed by its accumulation in the cytoplasm, migration to the nucleus, and ultimately inducing WNT target gene transcription. During embryogenesis, differentiation of chondrocytes from mesenchymal progenitors in the developing limb appears to be inhibited by the canonical WNT/β-catenin pathway, and may also require noncanonical WNT signaling. Later in embryonic development, both pathways appear to be needed for normal proliferation and differentiation of chondrocytes [48, 49]. High levels of WNT signaling in mesenchymal condensations can block chondrocyte differentiation and promote osteoblast differentiation directly into intramembranous ossification [48]. Conversely, conditional inactivation of β-catenin in undifferentiated mesenchymal cells results in ectopic chondrocyte formation with the absence of bone cells [50, 51]. Inactivation of β-catenin in murine embryonic chondrocytes decreased chondrocyte proliferation and hypertrophic differentiation [51, 52] Ablation of WNT-5a, acting through the noncanonical calcium pathway, results in decreased proliferation in the proliferative zone and delayed hypertrophic differentiation [53]. In addition to BMPs, FGFs and IHH/PTHrP, SOX9 also plays an important inhibiting role in WNT signaling of chondrogenesis. Co-transfection of mesenchymal progenitors in micro-mass cultures with WNT14, known to inhibit cartilage nodule formation, is rescued by SOX9 by enhancing β-catenin degradation [54].

Recent studies have revealed the importance of WNT/β-catenin signaling during postnatal growth. Conditional inhibition of WNT/β-catenin signaling in chondrocytes using transgenic mice expressing a dominant negative β-catenin under the collagen type 2 promoter results in postnatal survival of transgenic mice with normal birth size, followed by decreased skeletal growth, due to reduced chondrocyte proliferation and differentiation, an increase in chondrocyte apoptosis and delayed ossification [55]. Interestingly, transient activation of WNT/β-catenin signaling in young adult mice induces a somewhat similar phenotype with growth retardation, increased chondrocyte apoptosis, and abnormal growth plate closure [56].

WNT-2b, -4, and -10b, belonging to the canonical β-catenin pathway, and WNT-5a, -5b, and -11, which signal through the noncanonical calcium pathway, are expressed in the postnatal mouse growth plate [57]. Interestingly, these WNTs also show a remarkably similar expression pattern: low production in the resting zone, increasing WNT synthesis upon chondrocyte differentiation in the proliferative and prehypertrophic region, and decreased WNT expression in the hypertrophic zone. This overall gene expression pattern is broadly consistent with previous mouse embryo studies, suggesting that WNTs from the canonical as well as the noncanonical pathways modulate chondrocyte hypertrophic differentiation [57].

The roles of specific WNTs have been addressed in transgenic and gene targeting studies. Overexpression of WNT-4 accelerates chondrocyte hypertrophy [58]. However, mild or no growth phenotypes are observed for WNT-4 and WNT-10b knockout mice, in contrast with the more severely delayed hypertrophic differentiation as well as decreased chondrocyte proliferation in mice lacking β-catenin. This may be attributable to redundancy between these WNTs in growth plate chondrocytes [57].

In addition, the noncanonical calcium pathway, which antagonizes the canonical WNT/β-catenin pathway by promoting β-catenin degradation [59], appears to have an important role in growth plate formation and function. WNT-5a null mice display a severe skeletal phenotype with limb truncation and delayed chondrocyte hypertrophy, suggesting that WNT-5a promotes chondrocyte hypertrophy [53, 60]. In contrast, WNT-5b overexpression increases proliferative zone height presumably due to delayed cell cycle withdrawal and chondrocyte hypertrophy [53]. The finding that several members of the WNT family have similar expression patterns in the postnatal growth plate suggests that they may have overlapping or interacting roles in postnatal growth [57]. Therefore, ablation of these genes in combination may reveal a qualitative growth plate phenotype which is different from the ablation of any one of them alone. Eventually, these studies will give us new insights into the role of WNTs in pre- and postnatal growth.

Conclusions

Longitudinal bone growth is governed by a multitude of endocrine signals that interacts with a complex system of paracrine signals within the growth plate. Whereas knowledge of the endocrine systems involved in the regulation of longitudinal bone growth is fairly well understood, the complexity of the local regulation is just starting to unfold. New experimental approaches, including inducible and tissue-specific gene targeting, traditional and laser-assisted microdissection, microarray analysis, and linkage studies exploiting the full sequence of the human and mouse genomes have accelerated the progress in understanding the paracrine regulatory system as well as the precise interactions of endocrine and paracrine signals. These advances will eventually lead to improved understanding of human skeletal growth disorders and, combined with stem-cell biology and tissue engineering, are likely to yield new therapeutic approaches.

References

1 Kember NF: Cell population kinetics of bone growth: the first ten years of autoradiographic studies with tritiated thymidine. Clin Orthop Relat Res 1971;76:213–230.

2 Abad V, Meyers JL, Weise M, Gafni RI, Barnes KM, Nilsson O, Bacher JD, Baron J: The role of the resting zone in growth plate chondrogenesis. Endocrinology 2002;143:1851–1857.

3 Hunziker EB: Mechanism of longitudinal bone growth and its regulation by growth plate chondrocytes. Microsc Res Tech 1994;28:505–519.

4 Gerber HP, Vu TH, Ryan AM, Kowalski J, Werb Z, Ferrara N: VEGF couples hypertrophic cartilage remodeling, ossification and angiogenesis during endochondral bone formation. Nat Med 1999;5:623–628.

5 Farnum CE, Wilsman NJ: Cellular turnover at the chondro-osseous junction of growth plate cartilage: analysis by serial sections at the light microscopical level. J Orthop Res 1989;7:654–666.

6 Martin TJ, Moseley JM, Gillespie MT: Parathyroid hormone-related protein: Biochemistry and molecular biology. Crit Rev Biochem Mol Biol 1991;26:377–395.

7 Karaplis AC, Luz A, Glowacki J, Bronson RT, Tybulewicz VL, Kronenberg HM, Mulligan RC: Lethal skeletal dysplasia from targeted disruption of the parathyroid hormone-related peptide gene. Genes Dev 1994;8:277–289.

8 Lanske B, Karaplis AC, Lee K, Luz A, Vortkamp A, Pirro A, Karperien M, Defize LH, Ho C, Mulligan RC, Abou-Samra AB, Juppner H, Segre GV, Kronenberg HM: PTH/PTHrP receptor in early development and Indian hedgehog-regulated bone growth. Science 1996;273:663–666.

9 Weir EC, Philbrick WM, Amling M, Neff LA, Baron R, Broadus AE: Targeted overexpression of parathyroid hormone-related peptide in chondrocytes causes chondrodysplasia and delayed endochondral bone formation. Proc Natl Acad Sci USA 1996;93:10240–10245.

10 Chung UI, Lanske B, Lee K, Li E, Kronenberg H: The parathyroid hormone/parathyroid hormone-related peptide receptor coordinates endochondral bone development by directly controlling chondrocyte differentiation. Proc Natl Acad Sci U S A 1998;95:13030–13035.

11 Jobert AS, Zhang P, Couvineau A, Bonaventure J, Roume J, Le Merrer M, Silve C: Absence of functional receptors for parathyroid hormone and parathyroid hormone-related peptide in Blomstrand chondrodysplasia. J Clin Invest 1998;102:34–40.

12 Karaplis AC, He B, Nguyen MT, Young ID, Semeraro D, Ozawa H, Amizuka N: Inactivating mutation in the human parathyroid hormone receptor type 1 gene in blomstrand chondrodysplasia. Endocrinology 1998;139:5255–5258.

13 Schipani E, Langman CB, Parfitt AM, Jensen GS, Kikuchi S, Kooh SW, Cole WG, Juppner H: Constitutively activated receptors for parathyroid hormone and parathyroid hormone-related peptide in Jansen's metaphyseal chondrodysplasia. N Engl J Med 1996;335:708–714.

14 Lai LP, Mitchell J: Indian hedgehog: its roles and regulation in endochondral bone development. J Cell Biochem 2005;96:1163–1173.

15 Chung UI, Schipani E, McMahon AP, Kronenberg HM: Indian hedgehog couples chondrogenesis to osteogenesis in endochondral bone development. J Clin Invest 2001;107:295–304.

16 St-Jacques B, Hammerschmidt M, McMahon AP: Indian hedgehog signaling regulates proliferation and differentiation of chondrocytes and is essential for bone formation. Genes Dev 1999;13:2072–2086.

17 Vortkamp A, Pathi S, Peretti GM, Caruso EM, Zaleske DJ, Tabin CJ: Recapitulation of signals regulating embryonic bone formation during postnatal growth and in fracture repair. Mech Dev 1998;71:65–76.

18 Kobayashi T, Soegiarto DW, Yang Y, Lanske B, Schipani E, McMahon AP, Kronenberg HM: Indian hedgehog stimulates periarticular chondrocyte differentiation to regulate growth plate length independently of PTHrP. J Clin Invest 2005;115:1734–1742.

19 Vortkamp A, Lee K, Lanske B, Segre GV, Kronenberg HM, Tabin CJ: Regulation of rate of cartilage differentiation by Indian hedgehog and PTH-related protein. Science 1996;273:613–622.

20 Hogan BL: Bone morphogenetic proteins: multifunctional regulators of vertebrate development. Genes Dev 1996;10:1580–1594.

21 Koziel L, Wuelling M, Schneider S, Vortkamp A: Gli3 acts as a repressor downstream of Ihh in regulating two distinct steps of chondrocyte differentiation. Development 2005;132:5249–5260.

22 Hellemans J, Coucke PJ, Giedion A, De Paepe A, Kramer P, Beemer F, Mortier GR: Homozygous mutations in Ihh cause acrocapitofemoral dysplasia, an autosomal recessive disorder with cone-shaped epiphyses in hands and hips. Am J Hum Genet 2003;72:1040–1046.

23 Gao B, Hu J, Stricker S, Cheung M, Ma G, Law KF, Witte F, Briscoe J, Mundlos S, He L, Cheah KS, Chan D: A mutation in Ihh that causes digit abnormalities alters its signalling capacity and range. Nature 2009; 458:1196–1200.

24 Horton WA, Degnin CR: FGFs in endochondral skeletal development. Trends Endocrinol Metab 2009;20:341–348.

25 Mohammadi M, Olsen SK, Ibrahimi OA: Structural basis for fibroblast growth factor receptor activation. Cytokine Growth Factor Rev 2005;16:107–137.

26 Itoh N, Ornitz DM: Functional evolutionary history of the mouse Fgf gene family. Dev Dyn 2008;237: 18–27.

27 Peters K, Ornitz D, Werner S, Williams L: Unique expression pattern of the Fgf receptor 3 gene during mouse organogenesis. Dev Biol 1993;155:423–430.

28 Lazarus JE, Hegde A, Andrade AC, Nilsson O, Baron J: Fibroblast growth factor expression in the postnatal growth plate. Bone 2007;40:577–586.

29 Mason IJ, Fuller-Pace F, Smith R, Dickson C: Fgf-7 (keratinocyte growth factor) expression during mouse development suggests roles in myogenesis, forebrain regionalisation and epithelial-mesenchymal interactions. Mech Dev 1994;45:15–30.

30 Finch PW, Cunha GR, Rubin JS, Wong J, Ron D: Pattern of keratinocyte growth factor and keratinocyte growth factor receptor expression during mouse fetal development suggests a role in mediating morphogenetic mesenchymal-epithelial interactions. Dev Dyn 1995;203:223–240.

31 Xu J, Liu Z, Ornitz DM: Temporal and spatial gradients of Fgf8 and Fgf17 regulate proliferation and differentiation of midline cerebellar structures. Development 2000;127:1833–1843.

32 Liu Z, Xu J, Colvin JS, Ornitz DM: Coordination of chondrogenesis and osteogenesis by fibroblast growth factor 18. Genes Dev 2002;16:859–869.

33 Chen L, Adar R, Yang X, Monsonego EO, Li C, Hauschka PV, Yayon A, Deng CX: Gly369cys mutation in mouse Fgfr3 causes achondroplasia by affecting both chondrogenesis and osteogenesis. J Clin Invest 1999;104:1517–1525.

34 Colvin JS, Bohne BA, Harding GW, McEwen DG, Ornitz DM: Skeletal overgrowth and deafness in mice lacking fibroblast growth factor receptor 3. Nat Genet 1996;12:390–397.

35 Liu JP, Baker J, Perkins AS, Robertson EJ, Efstratiadis A: Mice carrying null mutations of the genes encoding insulin-like growth factor I (IGF-1) and type 1 IGF receptor (IGF1R). Cell 1993;75:59–72.

36 Brunet LJ, McMahon JA, McMahon AP, Harland RM: Noggin, cartilage morphogenesis, and joint formation in the mammalian skeleton. Science 1998;280:1455–1457.

37 Zhao GQ: Consequences of knocking out BMP signaling in the mouse. Genesis 2003;35:43–56.

38 Derynck R, Zhang YE: Smad-dependent and Smad-independent pathways in TGF-beta family signalling. Nature 2003;425:577–584.

39 Zou H, Wieser R, Massague J, Niswander L: Distinct roles of type I bone morphogenetic protein receptors in the formation and differentiation of cartilage. Genes Dev 1997;11:2191–2203.

40 Zou H, Niswander L: Requirement for BMP signaling in interdigital apoptosis and scale formation. Science 1996;272:738–741.

41 Khokha MK, Hsu D, Brunet LJ, Dionne MS, Harland RM: Gremlin is the BMP antagonist required for maintenance of Shh and Fgf signals during limb patterning. Nat Genet 2003;34:303–307

42 De Luca F, Barnes KM, Uyeda JA, De-Levi S, Abad V, Palese T, Mericq V, Baron J: Regulation of growth plate chondrogenesis by bone morphogenetic protein-2. Endocrinology 2001;142:430–436.

43 Kobayashi T, Lyons KM, McMahon AP, Kronenberg HM: BMP signaling stimulates cellular differentiation at multiple steps during cartilage development. Proc Natl Acad Sci U S A 2005;102:18023–18027.

44 Nilsson O, Parker EA, Hegde A, Chau M, Barnes KM, Baron J: Gradients in bone morphogenetic protein-related gene expression across the growth plate. J Endocrinol 2007;193:75–84.

45 Kawai S, Sugiura T: Characterization of human bone morphogenetic protein (BMP)-4 and -7 gene promoters: activation of BMP promoters by Gli, a sonic hedgehog mediator. Bone 2001;29:54–61.

46 Minina E, Kreschel C, Naski MC, Ornitz DM, Vortkamp A: Interaction of FGF, Ihh/Pthlh, and BMP signaling integrates chondrocyte proliferation and hypertrophic differentiation. Dev Cell 2002;3: 439–449.

47 Macsai CE, Foster BK, Xian CJ: Roles of Wnt signalling in bone growth, remodelling, skeletal disorders and fracture repair. J Cell Physiol 2008;215:578–587.
48 Day TF, Guo X, Garrett-Beal L, Yang Y: Wnt/beta-catenin signaling in mesenchymal progenitors controls osteoblast and chondrocyte differentiation during vertebrate skeletogenesis. Dev Cell 2005;8:739–750.
49 Yang Y: Wnts and wing: Wnt signaling in vertebrate limb development and musculoskeletal morphogenesis. Birth Defects Res C Embryo Today 2003;69:305–317.
50 Hu H, Hilton MJ, Tu X, Yu K, Ornitz DM, Long F: Sequential roles of hedgehog and wnt signaling in osteoblast development. Development 2005;132:49–60.
51 Hill TP, Spater D, Taketo MM, Birchmeier W, Hartmann C: Canonical Wnt/beta-catenin signaling prevents osteoblasts from differentiating into chondrocytes. Dev Cell 2005;8:727–738.
52 Akiyama H, Lyons JP, Mori-Akiyama Y, Yang X, Zhang R, Zhang Z, Deng JM, Taketo MM, Nakamura T, Behringer RR, McCrea PD, de Crombrugghe B: Interactions between SOX9 and beta-catenin control chondrocyte differentiation. Genes Dev 2004;18:1072–1087.
53 Yang Y, Topol L, Lee H, Wu J: Wnt5a and Wnt5b exhibit distinct activities in coordinating chondrocyte proliferation and differentiation. Development 2003;130:1003–1015.
54 Topol L, Chen W, Song H, Day TF, Yang Y: SOX9 inhibits Wnt signaling by promoting beta-catenin phosphorylation in the nucleus. J Biol Chem 2009;284:3323–3333.
55 Chen M, Zhu M, Awad H, Li TF, Sheu TJ, Boyce BF, Chen D, O'Keefe RJ: Inhibition of beta-catenin signaling causes defects in postnatal cartilage development. J Cell Sci 2008;121:1455–1465.
56 Yuasa T, Kondo N, Yasuhara R, Shimono K, Mackem S, Pacifici M, Iwamoto M, Enomoto-Iwamoto M: Transient activation of Wnt/beta-catenin signaling induces abnormal growth plate closure and articular cartilage thickening in postnatal mice. Am J Pathol 2009;175:1993–2003.
57 Andrade AC, Nilsson O, Barnes KM, Baron J: Wnt gene expression in the post-natal growth plate: regulation with chondrocyte differentiation. Bone 2007;40:1361–1369.
58 Hartmann C, Tabin CJ: Dual roles of Wnt signaling during chondrogenesis in the chicken limb. Development 2000;127:3141–3159.
59 Topol L, Jiang X, Choi H, Garrett-Beal L, Carolan PJ, Yang Y: Wnt-5a inhibits the canonical Wnt pathway by promoting GSK-3-independent beta-catenin degradation. J Cell Biol 2003;162:899–908.
60 Yamaguchi TP, Bradley A, McMahon AP, Jones S: A Wnt5a pathway underlies outgrowth of multiple structures in the vertebrate embryo. Development 1999;126:1211–1223.

Dr. Ola Nilsson
Center for Molecular Medicine and Pediatric Endocrinology Unit, Q2:08
Department of Women's and Children's Health, Karolinska Institutet and University Hospital
SE–171 76 Stockholm (Sweden)
Tel. +46 8 5177 9674, E-Mail ola.nilsson@ki.se

Camacho-Hübner C, Nilsson O, Sävendahl L (eds): Cartilage and Bone Development and Its Disorders.
Endocr Dev. Basel, Karger, 2011, vol 21, pp 23–29

Growth Plate Senescence and Catch-Up Growth

Julian C. Lui[a] · Ola Nilsson[b] · Jeffrey Baron[a]

[a]Developmental Endocrinology Branch, Program in Developmental Endocrinology and Genetics, Eunice Kennedy Shriver National Institute of Child Health and Human Development, National Institutes of Health, Bethesda, Md., USA; [b]Center for Molecular Medicine and Pediatric Endocrinology Unit Q2:08, Department of Women's and Children's Health, Karolinska Institutet and Karolinska University Hospital, Stockholm, Sweden

Abstract

Longitudinal bone growth is rapid in prenatal and early postnatal life, but then slows with age and eventually ceases. This growth deceleration is caused primarily by a decrease in chondrocyte proliferation, and is associated with other structural, functional, and molecular changes collectively termed growth plate senescence. Current evidence suggests that growth plate senescence occurs because the progenitor chondrocytes in the resting zone have a limited replicative capacity which is gradually exhausted with increasing cell division. In addition, recent experimental findings from laboratory and clinical studies suggest that growth plate senescence explains the phenomenon of catch-up growth. Growth-inhibiting conditions such as glucocorticoid excess and hypothyroidism delay the program of growth plate senescence. Consequently, growth plates are less senescent after these conditions resolve and therefore grow more rapidly than is normal for age, resulting in catch-up growth.

In humans, body length increases rapidly during fetal life and early childhood, but linear growth progressively slows and eventually ceases during adolescence. Similar declines in linear growth rates are also observed in other mammals. Although linear growth is highly regulated by endocrine factors, this decline in growth rate does not appear to be caused by a change in hormone levels. Indeed, there is no known growth-regulating hormone whose concentration changes in a pattern that would explain the slowing of linear growth. For example, circulating insulin-like growth factor-I concentrations rise during early childhood as growth is slowing [1]. Furthermore, growth plate transplantation experiments suggest that growth deceleration is not caused by any systemic mechanism; when growth plates are transplanted between rabbits of different ages, the growth rate of the transplanted growth plates depends on the age of the donor animal rather than the recipient [2], indicating that the decline in growth rate is primarily due to a mechanism intrinsic to the growth plates themselves.

The rate of longitudinal bone growth and hence the rate at which body length increases, is primarily determined by the rate of chondrocyte proliferation, the size attained by the hypertrophic chondrocytes, and the rate of cartilage matrix secretion [3]. In fact, the rate of longitudinal bone growth can be approximated mathematically by the number of cell divisions occurring in each proliferative column per unit time, multiplied by the height of the terminal hypertrophic chondrocyte [4]. This formula has a simple theoretical explanation; the number of cell divisions per column equals the number of new cells produced per unit time, and the height of the last hypertrophic chondrocyte approximates the amount of linear distance that will eventually be provided by each of those new cells. Cartilage matrix synthesis, while not explicitly part of the formula, is required to expand the intercolumnar extracellular space in the direction parallel to the long axis of the bone at a rate commensurate with that of the cellular expansion within the columns.

The decline in linear growth rate in the rat is due both to a decline in the proliferation rate and the size of the terminal hypertrophic cells [5, 6]. Of these, the greater fold change occurs in the rate of chondrocyte proliferation. Presumably, the rate of cartilage matrix synthesis is also declining to keep pace with the decline in cellular growth.

The progressive loss of function that occurs with increasing age in the growth plate is accompanied by a structural involution [6–8]. With increasing age, the overall height of the growth plate declines because of a decrease in the number of resting zone chondrocytes and the number of proliferative and hypertrophic chondrocytes per column. In addition, the columns of chondrocytes become more widely spaced with age. These senescent structural changes have been best studied in rodents and rabbits. In humans, the rate of longitudinal growth also declines with age, as do both the number of chondrocytes per cell column [9, 10] and the proportion of proliferative chondrocytes per column [9]. However, unlike rats, the height of the terminal hypertrophic cells and the height of the resting zone in human growth plates remain relatively constant during the period of juvenile growth deceleration [10].

This postnatal development program, which includes both progressive loss of function and progressive structural involution, has been termed growth plate senescence [11, 12]. In biology, the word senescence has two meanings [13]. First, it can refer to physiological changes that occur with increasing age and typically involve a loss of function. Second, the word can refer to a specific cellular program that was first identified in cultured cells and includes a cessation in proliferation [13]. The term growth plate senescence uses the first meaning and simply refers to a physiological program that involves a loss of function and involution with increasing age.

The fact that growth plate senescence occurs with increasing age suggests the possibility that senescence is driven by a timing mechanism within the growth plate, such as a biological clock; however, several studies indicate that this is not the case. Conditions that slow growth in the growth plate also slow the entire development program of growth plate senescence, suggesting that the process of growth, rather than age per se, is the underlying driver of senescence. The specific experimental evidence for this conclusion comes from several animal models including growth inhibition by glucocorticoid excess in the rabbit [12], inhibition by hypothyroidism in rats [7], and inhibition by tryptophan deficiency (and consequently decreased food intake) in rats [unpubl. obs.]. In each system, the experimental intervention slows longitudinal bone growth and also slows the changes in structural and functional markers of growth plate senescence. These observations that slowing growth using multiple different approaches slows senescence strongly imply that senescence is a function of growth rather than simply a function of age. However, the data do not exclude the possibility that age itself may also play some contributory role. How might growth drive senescence? One possibility is that chondrocytes might have some mechanisms to count cell cycles. Such cell-cycle counting appears to occur in some developmental processes. For example, the *Xenopus laevis* embryo undergoes exactly twelve synchronous cleavages before a period of slower asynchronous cell divisions [14]. This putative cell cycle counter in growth plate chondrocytes could involve some characteristic of the cell that is progressively altered with each cell division. As the cumulative number of cell divisions undergone increases, this putative counter might advance and then turn off growth-promoting factors and/or turn on growth-inhibiting factors, causing proliferation to slow.

Whether or not a cell-cycle counter exists in the growth plate, it appears likely that the growth plate retains information about its prior growth history and that this prior growth history affects future growth. Theoretical considerations suggest that this information about the prior growth history is not stored in the proliferative or hypertrophic zone. The hypertrophic chondrocytes undergo apoptosis and are soon lost from the growth plate. The proliferative chondrocytes undergo clonal expansion briefly but are not thought to be self-renewing but rather undergo terminal differentiation to become hypertrophic chondrocytes and thus are subsequently lost to apoptosis. One could imagine that the information regarding prior growth history is somehow stored in these zones but passed on to surrounding cells so that it is not lost as each cell dies. However, another simpler explanation is that the prior growth history is retained in the resting zone. This zone appears to contain progenitor chondrocytes that can produce new columnar clones of proliferative and hypertrophic chondrocytes and are thought to persist, self-renewing by slow cell division, throughout the lifespan of the growth plate [15]. If this slow replication of progenitor cells in the resting zone were to gradually deplete their replicative capacity, then their clonal progeny in the proliferative zone might also show progressively diminished proliferative activity, leading to growth deceleration. Alternatively, if the progenitor cells were simply to become depleted numerically, the proliferative columns might be renewed less often. This might account for the decrease in column density that occurs with senescence as well as the decrease in proliferation within each column. In fact, there is evidence that the resting zone chondrocytes do become depleted both in number and proliferative activity as senescence progresses [16]. This qualitative and quantitative depletion might be interrelated; a loss of proliferative capacity in these cells might limit not only their ability to generate active proliferative clones but also their ability to self-renew, leading to their own numerical depletion. Interestingly, treatment with glucocorticoid excess in vivo slows chondrocyte proliferation in the resting zone and also slows the numerical depletion of these cells, consistent with the hypothesis that the numerical depletion of these cells is dependent on the cumulative number of cell divisions undergone [16].

Although the proliferative activity of resting zone chondrocytes declines during senescence in vivo, this decline may not necessarily be due to a cell-autonomous depletion of proliferative capacity. When resting zone chondrocytes are isolated from rabbits and cultured in vitro, they undergo a limited number of cell divisions before undergoing replicative senescence. However, the number of population doublings that these cells undergo seems to be fixed rather than dependent on whether the cells were obtained from fetal rabbits, rapidly growing young rabbits, or older rabbits that grow more slowly [17]. This finding suggests that the mechanisms responsible for limiting proliferation in vivo and the mechanisms that limit proliferation in cell culture are different. This observation also raises the possibility that the mechanisms limiting growth in vivo are not cell autonomous but rather require cell-cell interaction. As an example, slowing of proliferation might reflect decreasing expression of a paracrine growth factor. When cells are taken from the growth plate and placed in culture, their growth may no longer be limited by this factor but rather by growth factors added to the culture medium, allowing them to bypass the in vivo limit and continue growing until they reach a different limit, perhaps the same limit that prevents other cell types from growing indefinitely when placed in culture, the Hayflick limit [18].

The molecular mechanisms that slow growth in vivo are not well understood. However, recent studies suggest that there is a complex set of changes in gene expression that occurs in the growth plate during senescence that may contribute to this developmental process. Gene expression has been assessed in young rats, which are growing rapidly, and older rats, which are growing more slowly [19]. This comparison was done by microdissecting the proliferative plus early hypertrophic zone from these rats, isolating RNA and then measuring specific mRNA levels by expression microarray analysis, followed by verification using real-time RT-PCR. This analysis has pointed to specific candidate genes, such as *Igf2*, a growth-promoting gene which is downregulated almost 1,000-fold during senescence [20]. This analysis also suggests that FGF, WNT, eicosanoid, p38-MAPK and vitamin D receptor signaling may be involved [19, 21]. There is evidence that the decline in *Igf2* mRNA expression and a limited number of other changes in expression are driven by growth, rather than by time, suggesting that these changes are part of the senescence program [7]. Nevertheless, substantial additional investigation will be required to test whether these pathways are only temporally associated with growth plate senescence or they indeed play a causal role.

Our improved understanding of growth plate senescence has provided insight into the clinical phenomenon of catch-up growth. Catch-up growth is defined as body growth that occurs at a rate greater than normal for age, following a period of growth inhibition [22]. Clinically, catch-up growth has been observed after growth inhibition due to a variety of causes, including hypothyroidism, malnutrition, and glucocorticoid excess. Previously, catch-up growth was ascribed to a homeostatic mechanism within the central nervous system [23]. However, local growth inhibition within a single growth plate leads to local catch-up growth, suggesting that the mechanism responsible for catch-up growth resides, at least in part, within the growth plates themselves [24]. Subsequent studies have shown evidence that this local catch-up growth results from delayed growth plate senescence. Growth-inhibiting conditions slow senescence, including the decline in the chondrocyte proliferation rate, the size of the hypertrophic chondrocyte and, consequently, the rate of longitudinal bone growth [7, 12]. Therefore, when the growth-inhibiting condition resolves, the growth plates grow more rapidly than is normal for age, resulting in catch-up growth. Simply put, because growth-inhibiting conditions slow aging of the growth plate, after the condition resolves, the growth plates grow more rapidly like those of younger animals. The evidence for this mechanism comes from studies of catch-up growth after glucocorticoid excess in rabbits [12] and after hypothyroidism in rats [7].

Indirect evidence suggests that catch-up growth in humans is also due to delayed growth plate senescence. In children with celiac disease, growth is often inhibited, and, when a gluten-free diet is initiated, catch-up growth occurs. In these children, the rate of growth during the first 4 years of treatment was greater than expected for age (indicating catch-up growth) but normal for a younger child, based on their height age or bone age at the time of treatment initiation [25]. This pattern of right shift in the growth curve during catch-up growth was consistent with the hypothesis that delayed senescence contributes to catch-up growth.

In summary, with increasing age, the growth plate undergoes programmed senescence, including both loss of function and structural involution. Growth plate senescence appears to be driven not by time, which would suggest a biological clock mechanism, but by growth itself, suggesting the possibility of a cell-cycle counting mechanism. Theoretical considerations and limited empirical findings suggest that the information about the prior growth history is stored in the resting zone. The stem-like cells in this zone appear to be depleted during senescence, both quantitatively and also qualitatively, in terms of their proliferative activity. The molecular mechanisms that cause growth plate senescence are not well understood, but may involve a complex set of changes in gene expression that occurs in the growth plate postnatally. Finally, growth plate senescence appears to explain an interesting clinical phenomenon; there is evidence that catch-up growth is due to delayed growth plate senescence.

Acknowledgments

This work was supported by the Intramural Research Program of the Eunice Kennedy Shriver National Institute of Child Health and Human Development, NIH.

References

1 Zapf J, Walter H, Froesch ER: Radioimmunological determination of insulinlike growth factors I and II in normal subjects and in patients with growth disorders and extrapancreatic tumor hypoglycemia. J Clin Invest 1981;68:1321.

2 Stevens DG, Boyer MI, Bowen CV: Transplantation of epiphyseal plate allografts between animals of different ages. J Pediatr Orthop 1999;19:398.

3 Hunziker EB: Mechanism of longitudinal bone growth and its regulation by growth plate chondrocytes. Microsc Res Tech 1994;28:505.

4 Sissons HA: Experimental study on the effect of local radiation on bone growth; in Mitchell JS, Holmes BE, Smith CL (eds): Progress in Radiobiology. Edinburgh, Oliver and Boyd, 1955, pp 436–452.

5 Kember NF, Walker KV: Control of bone growth in rats. Nature 1971;229:428.

6 Walker KV, Kember NF: Cell kinetics of growth cartilage in the rat tibia. II. Measurements during ageing. Cell Tissue Kinet 1972;5:409.

7 Marino R, Hegde A, Barnes KM, Schrier L, Emons JA, Nilsson O, Baron J: Catch-up growth after hypothyroidism is caused by delayed growth plate senescence. Endocrinology 2008;149:1820.

8 Weise M, De-Levi S, Barnes KM, Gafni RI, Abad V, Baron J: Effects of estrogen on growth plate senescence and epiphyseal fusion. Proc Natl Acad Sci USA 2001;98:6871.

9 Sissons HA, Kember NF: Longitudinal bone growth of the human femur. Postgrad Med J 1977;53:433.

10 Kember NF, Sissons HA: Quantitative histology of the human growth plate. J Bone Joint Surg Br 1976; 58-B:426.

11 Nilsson O, Baron J: Fundamental limits on longitudinal bone growth: growth plate senescence and epiphyseal fusion. Trends Endocrinol Metab 2004; 15:370.

12 Gafni RI, Weise M, Robrecht DT, Meyers JL, Barnes KM, De-Levi S, Baron J: Catch-up growth is associated with delayed senescence of the growth plate in rabbits. Pediatr Res 2001;50:618.

13 Campisi J, d'Adda di Fagagna F: Cellular senescence: when bad things happen to good cells. Nat Rev Mol Cell Biol 2007;8:729.

14 Newport JW, Kirschner MW: Regulation of the cell cycle during early *Xenopus* development. Cell 1984; 37:731.

15 Abad V, Meyers JL, Weise M, Gafni RI, Barnes KM, Nilsson O, Bacher JD, Baron J: The role of the resting zone in growth plate chondrogenesis. Endocrinology 2002;143:1851.

16 Schrier L, Ferns SP, Barnes KM, Emons JA, Newman EI, Nilsson O, Baron J: Depletion of resting zone chondrocytes during growth plate senescence. J Endocrinol 2006;189:27.

17 Nilsson O, Mitchum RD Jr, Schrier L, Ferns SP, Barnes KM, Troendle JF, Baron J: Growth plate senescence is associated with loss of DNA methylation. J Endocrinol 2005;186:241.

18 Hayflick L: The limited in vitro lifetime of human diploid cell strains. Exp Cell Res 1965;37:614.

19 Lui JC, Andrade AC, Forcinito P, Hegde A, Chen W, Baron J, Nilsson O: Spatial and temporal regulation of gene expression in the mammalian growth plate. Bone 2010;46:1380.

20 Parker EA, Hegde A, Buckley M, Barnes KM, Baron J, Nilsson O: Spatial and temporal regulation of GH-IGF-related gene expression in growth plate cartilage. J Endocrinol 2007;194:31.

21 Lazarus JE, Hegde A, Andrade AC, Nilsson O, Baron J: Fibroblast growth factor expression in the postnatal growth plate. Bone 2007;40:577.

22 Boersma B, Wit JM: Catch-up growth. Endocr Rev 1997;18:646.

23 Tanner JM: Regulation of growth in size in mammals. Nature 1963;199:845.
24 Baron J, Klein KO, Colli MJ, Yanovski JA, Novosad JA, Bacher JD, Cutler GB Jr: Catch-up growth after glucocorticoid excess: a mechanism intrinsic to the growth plate. Endocrinology 1994;135:1367.
25 Emons JA, Boersma B, Baron J, Wit JM: Catch-up growth: testing the hypothesis of delayed growth plate senescence in humans. J Pediatr 2005;147:843.

Dr. Jeffrey Baron
National Institutes of Health, CRC, Room 1-3330
10 Center Drive, MSC-1103
Bethesda, MD 20892-1103 (USA)
Tel. +1 301 496 6312, Fax +1 301 402 0574, E-Mail jeffrey.baron@nih.gov

Camacho-Hübner C, Nilsson O, Sävendahl L (eds): Cartilage and Bone Development and Its Disorders.
Endocr Dev. Basel, Karger, 2011, vol 21, pp 30–41

Endocrine Regulation of Longitudinal Bone Growth

Jan M. Wit[a] · Cecilia Camacho-Hübner[b,c]

[a]Department of Paediatrics, Leiden University Medical Center, Leiden, The Netherlands; [b]Division of Pediatric Endocrinology, Department of Women's and Children's Health, Karolinska Institutet, Stockholm, Sweden, and [c]Pfizer Global Pharmaceuticals, New York, N.Y., USA

Abstract

Longitudinal growth is primarily influenced by the GH-IGF-I axis, which is a mixed endocrine-paracrine-autocrine system. Further, classical hormones such as thyroxine, glucocorticosteroids and sex steroids play a role, as well as primarily paracrine systems. In the GH-IGF-I axis, seven disorders can be differentiated: (1) GH deficiency; (2) *GHR* defects; (3) defects in the GH signal transduction pathway; (4) *IGF1* defects; (5) *IGFALS* defects; (6) *IGF1R* defects, and (7) *IGF2* defects. Children with one of the first 3 disorders have near-normal prenatal growth, while children with defects of *IGF1*, *IGF1R* or *IGF2* show prenatal as well as postnatal growth retardation. Hypothyroidism or a thyroid hormone resistance cause growth failure, but the effect of hyperthyroidism on growth is modest. Hypercortisolism causes poor growth, while FGD caused by ACTH insensitivity is associated with tall stature. Increased sex steroids in childhood cause advanced growth but even more skeletal maturation, so that adult height is decreased. Finally, the paracrine-autocrine SHOX-BNP pathway and the related CNP-NPR2 pathway are also involved in growth, as very many other growth factors and their receptors and mediators.

Most classifications of growth failure are based on the concept that there are disorders of the growth plate itself, usually termed primary growth failure, and of the milieu of the growth plate, usually termed secondary growth failure. The milieu can be abnormal in the sense of deficiencies, such as unavailability of sufficient oxygen, nutrients, and hormones, and in the sense of toxicity, such as increased concentrations of metabolic waste products (e.g. in renal, hepatic and metabolic disorders), toxins, interleukins, and various iatrogenic interventions (e.g. glucocorticosteroids, chemotherapy, irradiation). Psychosocial causes of growth failure, including psychosocial deprivation, anorexia nervosa and depression, are usually also classified under secondary growth failure as a separate category, although there are some indications that the effect of these conditions may be mediated via endocrine mechanisms. The third category of growth failure is termed 'idiopathic short stature', including familial and nonfamilial short stature.

The most frequently encountered category of secondary growth failure in affluent countries consists of endocrine disorders, including GH deficiency, hypothyroidism, and (more rarely) hypercortisolism (Cushing syndrome). Poor growth in poorly controlled diabetes and insulin resistance (leprechaunism) can also be categorized in this group, although the former can also be considered as an example of increased metabolic waste products. The effects of sex steroids on growth are more complex. Elevated levels of androgens or estrogens in infancy or childhood cause increased growth, but skeletal maturation is even more increased, so that adult height is decreased. On the other hand, a deficiency of sex steroids, such as in hypogonadism, causes a mild growth deceleration in adolescence, but adult height may be increased, with eunuchoidal body proportions, because of late growth plate closure.

While GH deficiency, hypothyroidism and hypercortisolism are endocrine disorders in the classical sense, downstream disorders in the GH-IGF-I axis are examples of the extended concept of endocrinology, encompassing paracrine and autocrine effects besides endocrine effects.

In this review, we shall primarily focus on the role of the various elements of the GH-IGF-I axis, as can be deducted from defects of the various genes involved. The role of thyroxine, glucocorticosteroids and sex steroids, as well as a primarily paracrine system encompassing SHOX/BNP and CNP and its receptor, will be discussed only shortly. We also focus primarily on postnatal growth. The role of the mother, placenta and fetus in endocrine regulation of human fetal growth has been recently reviewed by others [1].

The GH-IGF-I Axis

The GH-IGF-I axis is a complex system, in which various proteins play a role, with endocrine, paracrine and autocrine functions. Since the discovery of IGF-I (originally termed sulphation factor and then somatomedin), several hypotheses have been proposed about the function of this system. The so-called 'Somatomedin hypothesis' has been revised and revisited several times. Evidence generated in recent years suggests that the growth-promoting effects of GH may not be entirely mediated by circulating IGF-I, as was proposed in the original somatomedin hypothesis, and that paracrine/autocrine IGF-I activity may be significantly involved in this process [2].

Pituitary GH secretion, which is regulated by stimulatory (GHRH) and inhibitory (somatostatin) hypothalamic hormones, has a direct as well as indirect action on many tissues. One of the direct actions is to stimulate IGF-I, IGFBP-3 and the ALS, primarily from the liver, but GH also affects transcription of numerous other genes.

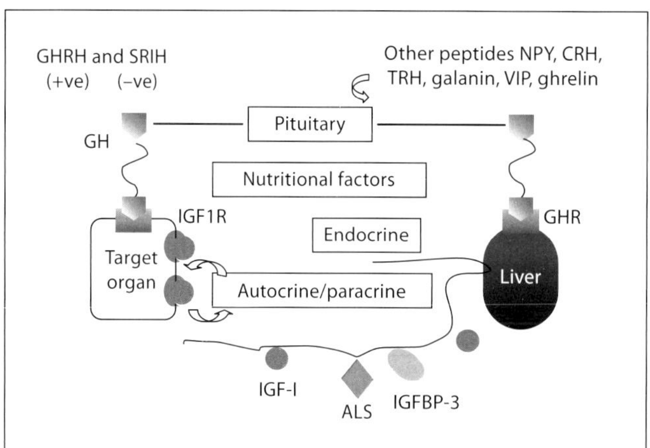

Fig. 1. Schematic representation of the neuroendocrine regulation of growth. Pituitary GH secretion is primarily controlled by two hypothalamic factors: GHRH, which has a stimulatory effect, and SRIH (also called somatostatin), which has an inhibitory effect. However, also other peptides have an effect on GH secretion, such as NPY, CRH, TRH, galanin, VIP and ghrelin. Circulatory GH is bound to receptors present in many tissues, and leads to the transcription of many target genes, including *IGF1*. At the local level, IGF-I has an autocrine and paracrine function. Circulating IGF-I, IGFBP-3 and ALS are primarily derived from the liver, and the major part of circulating IGF-I is bound to GHBP-3 and ALS.

Circulating IGF-I is primarily produced by the liver (under the influence of GH and other factors), and it is accepted that it acts primarily in an endocrine fashion. Most of circulating IGF-I is found as part of the 150-kDa ternary complex also containing its predominant IGF-binding proteins, IGFBP-3 and ALS (fig. 1).

A recent study on bi-transgenic mice carrying in an *Igf1* null background a dormant *Igf1* cDNA placed downstream of a transcriptional 'stop' DNA sequence flanked by *loxP* sites (floxed) and also a *cre* transgene driven by a liver-specific promoter showed that the endocrine IGF-I plays a significant role in mouse growth, as its action contributes to approximately 30% of the adult body size and sustains postnatal development, including the reproductive functions of both sexes in the mouse [3].

Traditionally, disorders in this axis have been classified according to the GH status: GH deficiency or GH insensitivity. More recently, some investigators have proposed to give IGF-I a more central role in the classification, and to distinguish secondary IGF deficiency (equal to GH deficiency, or other conditions causing low circulating IGF-I levels), primary IGF deficiency (all congenital forms of GH insensitivity; acquired GH insensitivity, for example because of malnutrition is called 'secondary'), and IGF resistance.

At present, there are five conditions associated with a low IGF-I in spite of a normal or elevated GH secretion: defects of *GHR*, *STAT5B*, *IKBKB (IκB)*, *IGF1* and *IGFALS*. The first of these is GH insensitivity syndrome or Laron syndrome caused by a homozygous defect of the *GHR*. This condition can still be seen as a disturbance in a classical endocrine feedback loop. Defects of the GHR signal transduction pathway (*STAT5B* or *IKBKB* defects) are different because these defects also have an impact on other biological pathways, such as interleukins. The effects of *IGF1* defects cannot be understood in the context of a pure 'classical' endocrine pathway: IGF-I is produced in virtually all cells of the body, and the local effects are more important for growth than the endocrine effects. Here also a time component comes into play: in utero, the IGF-I production is GH independent and mainly dependent of nutrition and insulin, but postnatally the IGF-I production is mainly dependent on GH-secretion, although nutrition and insulin secretion still play a role. Heterozygous defects of *IGF1R* cause a partial insensitivity to IGF-I, which apparently cannot be compensated by increased IGF-I production. The clinical presentation of children with an isolated *IGF2* defect is still uncertain.

We prefer to divide disorders of the GH-IGF-I axis into seven groups: (a) GH deficiency; (b) *GHR* defects; (c) defects in the GH signal transduction pathway; (d) *IGF1* defects; (e) *IGFALS* defects; (f) *IGF1R* defects; (g) *IGF2* defects.

GH Deficiency

The essential role of GH in growth is shown by patients with a total absence of pituitary GH secretion, for example children with a *GH1* gene deletion. Birth weight and length is usually in the normal range, but on average slightly decreased. It is estimated that the adult height loss in such conditions is approximately 4.7 SD (range –3.9 to –6.1 SDS in the four available studies) in patients with spontaneous puberty, and 3 SD if puberty is induced at an advanced age [4]. In cases with untreated hypogonadism, as part of multiple pituitary deficiency, adult height can even be normal or increased, due to extremely late closure of epiphyseal plates. Head circumference is usually normal. The role of GH is further substantiated by the observation that GH administration improves growth rate, and if started early enough and at an appropriate dosage, normalizes adult height [4]. GH deficiency either isolated or as part of multiple pituitary deficiency, can be caused by defects in several genes, which have been recently summarized [5].

GHR Defects

Laron syndrome, also called classical GH insensitivity, is a fully penetrant autosomal recessive disease, first described in 1966. To date, more than 250 patients have been described worldwide with 60 different mutations [6]. Mean birth length has been reported as –1 SDS in the European and Ecuadorian cohorts, but lower in Israeli patients, indicating that in late pregnancy there is already some dependency on GH.

Postnatal growth rate fails immediately after birth, and adult height is 139 and 123 cm for men and women, respectively [6], and head circumference is usually normal, similar to cases with complete GH deficiency [7].

Biochemically, GHBP is undetectable (table 1) or low in patients with extracellular domain mutations or deletions, while it can be normal or even increased in mutations in the part of the gene coding for the anchoring site or the intracellular part of the protein [7, 8]. Circulating IGF-I, IGFBP-3 and ALS are low, and IGFBP-1 and -2 can be increased. For further details on the clinical and biochemical presentation, the reader is referred to Mehta et al. [6]. A summary of the clinical and biochemical characteristics of cases with *GHR*, *STAT5B*, *IKBKB*, *IGF1*, *IGFALS* and *IGF1R* defects is presented in table 1.

Defects in the GH Signal Transduction Pathway

After binding of GH to its receptor, the signal has to be transferred to the cell nucleus to initiate gene transcription of several GH-dependent genes, particularly *IGF1*, *IGFBP3* and *IGFALS*. After GH, which is preformed as a dimer, binds to its receptor, a conformational change occurs, whereby JAK2 is autophosphorylated and activated, in turn leading to phosphorylation of STAT5a and STAT5b molecules. Phosphorylated STAT5 molecules dimerize and translocate to the nucleus, where they bind to DNA and activate target genes [6].

From in vitro investigations on the GH signal transduction pathway and animal studies, it was expected that *STAT5b* defects would lead to GH resistance, and indeed 7 families have been described in which homozygous defects of the *STAT5b* gene were encountered [8, 9]. Patients with homozygous *STAT5b* defects present with severe GH resistance and growth failure (height between –5.6 to –9.9 SDS), but a normal head circumference (–1.4 SDS; table 1). In all cases except one, this is also combined with a severe immune disorder [8], usually leading to pulmonary fibrosis, which is possibly explained by the role of STAT5B as a mediator of IL-2 action and T cell function. Circulating GH can be elevated, but in some cases a normal GH secretion was observed. An elevated serum prolactin has been found in most cases. Preliminary data suggest that a heterozygous defect may lead to a mild decrease in height SDS.

The GH signal transduction pathway is far more complex than a single straight line from GHR to JAK2, STAT5B and gene transcription. There appears to be much cross-talk between various proteins involved in different signal transduction pathways. An example of this is the observation that activating mutations of *PTPN11* (as seen in Noonan syndrome), leading to overactive SHP2, enhances RAS/MAPK signaling, but is associated in some cases with partial GH insensitivity. Similar phenotypes are observed in children with defects in other genes (SOS1 and KRAS) in the RAS/MAPK pathway, which give rise to several syndromes (e.g. Costello syndrome). Height is

Table 1. Clinical and biochemical characteristics of defects of the GH-IGF-I axis

	GHR–/–	STAT5B–/–	Ras-raf+/–	IKBKB+/–	IGFALS–/–	IGF1–/–	IGF1R+/–
Birth size SDS	N or mildly affected	N	N	N	N or low	–5.5 to –2.4	–4 to –1.5
Height SDS	–5.6 to –9.9 SDS	–4.9 to –9.9 SDS	–4 to –1 SDS	–4 SDS	–4.2 to –0.5	–6.9 to –8.5	–5.0 to –2.6
HC SDS	N	N	N or low	N	N or low	–8.0 to –4.0	–4 to –2
Parental height	N	N (1 SD lower than WT)	one parent may be affected	one parent may be affected	N (1 SD lower than WT)	N (1 SD lower than WT)	one parent may be affected
Clinical features	hypoglycemia; frontal bossing; midfacies hypoplasia	immuno-deficiency; pulmonary fibrosis; arthritis	dysmorphisms; pulmonary stenosis; in 40% mild mental handicap	mental retardation; leukocytosis	delayed puberty in 50% of males	mental retardation; deaf; pubertal delay	poor appetite; may be associated with defects of nervous and cardiac system
GHmax	⇑	⇑	N	⇑	N or ⇑	⇑	N or ⇑
IGF-I	⇓⇓	⇓⇓	⇓	⇓	⇓⇓	undetectable, low, or high	>0 SDS
IGFBP-3	⇓⇓	⇓⇓	N	⇓	⇓⇓⇓	N	N
ALS	⇓⇓	⇓⇓	⇓	?	undetectable	N	N
Other biochemical features	complete GH insensitivity; GHBP often undetectable; PRL N or slightly ⇑	(almost) complete GH insensitivity; PRL 61–169 ng/ml (N in one case)	partial GH insensitivity (variable)	hyper-IgM syndrome; immuno-deficiency	complete GH insensitivity	insulin resistance	on GH treatment strongly elevated IGF-I

HC = Head circumference; –/– = homozygous; +/– = heterozygous; N = normal; SDS = standard deviation score; WT = wild type; PRL = prolactin.

approximately 30 cm below the population's average [10] (table 1). Preliminary data suggest that haploinsufficiency of NSD1, a cause of Sotos syndrome which is associated with tall stature, may lead to suppression of the RAS/MAPK pathway [Visser et al., submitted].

Another gene which may be associated with a combination of GH resistance and immunodeficiency is *IKBKB (IκB)*. A heterozygous mutation of this gene was found in two unrelated cases with serious immune problems and short stature. We reported that one of these patients had severe short stature and GH resistance (table 1) [11]. The father of the patient, who was mosaic for the mutation, was also short, had a low serum IGF-I and experienced a mild immune problem in childhood.

IGF1 Defects

Homozygous *IGF1* defects are presumably very rare. After the first report of a homozygous deletion of IGF1 exons 4 and 5 [12], a family with 2 affected siblings with a homozygous missense mutation was identified [13], and recently a less severely affected third case was reported [14]. There may be a fourth case, but although the phenotype was very similar, the presumed genetic aberration at the polyadenylation site at the 3′UTR in exon 6 was later found to occur in healthy controls. Intrauterine growth is severely affected (about –4 SDS), height SDS is between –6.9 and –8.5, and head circumference between –8.0 and –4 SDS (table 1). Heterozygosity for an *IGF1* mutation or deletion may be associated with a mild height loss (in the order of 1 SD), which can present as short stature if occurring in a genetically short family [12, 13].

IGFALS Defects

As discussed earlier, local IGF-I appears more important for growth than circulating IGF-I. This was primarily noted in experimental animals, but since the discovery of patients with homozygous *IGFALS* mutations, it is clear that this also applies to the human. Homozygous *IGFALS* defects are associated with a modest height deficit (approximately –4.2 to –0.5 SDS), and in fact the first published case was short in childhood and adolescence, but had a normal adult height. A full description of this clinical syndrome was recently published [15], and a summary is presented in table 1. Heterozygosity for an *IGFALS* defect appears to lead to a 1 SD loss of height, which can also cause short stature in a family with a short genetic background [15].

IGF1R Defects

At present, the only known cause of IGF-I resistance is a heterozygous (or compound heterozygous) defect (mutation or deletion) of the *IGF1R* [16]. In a substantial part of the cases with an *IGF1R* defect, this is part of a larger deletion of the terminal region of 15q. Major criteria include a small birth size, short stature (approximately –5.0 to –2.6 SDS), small head circumference, and IGF-I >+0 SDS. In cases of a terminal chromosome 15q deletion, developmental delay and cardiac abnormalities can be seen. In our series, *IGF1R* defects were seen in 2% of short children born SGA [17]. It is highly likely that there may be disorders in the IGF-I signal transduction pathway, which also may be associated with short stature. However, so far these have not yet been discovered in the human.

IGF2 Defects

With respect to *IGF2*, as far as we know 2 patients have been described in whom pre- and postnatal growth retardation was associated with a balanced chromosomal translocation of paternal origin, disrupting the regulatory region of the *IGF2* gene [18]. No mutations or deletions have yet been reported. Imprinting disorders of 11p15 (including *IGF2*) cause Russell-Silver syndrome, but also other genetic defects are associated with this syndrome [19].

Thyroxine

There are two thyroid conditions associated with short stature: hypothyroidism and thyroid hormone resistance. Primary congenital hypothyroidism, due to thyroid agenesis or dysgenesis, or an inborn error of thyroid hormonogenesis, is inevitably associated with severe growth failure, which is even more extreme than observed in GH deficiency. Such extreme cases of cretinism are now only seen in countries with severely deficient medical care, or in cases where parents hid the patient from medical attention [20]. Treatment with L-thyroxine causes a dramatic rise in growth velocity, but adult height is still decreased. Also acquired hypothyroidism, usually due to Hashimoto thyroiditis, causes growth failure. L-thyroxine treatment restores growth velocity, but adult height may still be lower than target height [21].

Thyroid hormone resistance is characterized by poor growth, hyperactivity, learning disability or other nonspecific signs or symptoms. A small goiter may also be present. It is usually caused by a point mutation in the hinge region or ligand-binding domain of the *THRB* gene.

The effect of hyperthyroidism, as seen in Graves's disease, on growth is less clear. Acceleration of linear growth may occur, but is often accompanied by advanced skeletal maturation. It is generally assumed that adult height is not affected.

Glucocorticoids

Under normal circumstances, glucocorticoids play a minor role in growth regulation. Glucocorticoids have a direct effect on growth through their receptors that are present on virtually all cells including chondrocytes in the growth plate. In addition, glucocorticoid treatment has a biphasic effect on GH secretion: an initial acute stimulation within 3 h, followed by suppression within 12 h. The latter is a clinically important effect, as excess of endogenous and exogenous glucocorticoids is well known to suppress growth in children [22].

Low cortisol levels have no effect on growth, except for one condition: FGD caused by ACTH insensitivity. This syndrome is also called hereditary unresponsiveness to ACTH, and is associated with tall stature. There are at least two forms of this disorder: FGD1 (25%) caused by mutations in the ACTH receptor (FGD1) and FGD2 caused by mutations in the gene encoding the MRAP (20%). Thus, for 55% of the cases, no genetic cause has yet been found [23].

Androgens

The effect of androgens on growth has not been fully clarified. Arguments in favor of a direct effect of androgens are the presence of androgen receptors in the growth plate, expanding width of the growth plate after injecting testosterone into the growth plate, and the growth acceleration in children on treatment with nonaromatizable androgens [for review, see 24]. However, there are more arguments in favor of the hypothesis that the main effect of androgens is obtained through conversion to estrogens, by local aromatase [25]. This is supported by observations in men with aromatase deficiency who presented with delayed bone development and osteopenia [26].

Estrogens

Estrogens play an important role in growth regulation, both directly and indirectly (through interaction with the GH-IGF-I axis), not only in females but also in males. However, the effect is biphasic, low concentrations stimulating growth and higher concentrations leading to decreasing and finally cessation of growth [27]. A further complicating factor is that estrogens have a strong influence on skeletal maturation, and are necessary for epiphyseal closure [28]. In the male, estrogens are mainly produced intracellularly by aromatase that is present in many cell types, including chondrocytes in the growth plate [25]. The local effects are discussed in another chapter of this volume.

Estrogens have a stimulatory effect on GH secretion. Increasing estrogen production in puberty, either produced by the ovaries in girls or by conversion from androgens in boys, increases the amplitude of spontaneous GH secretion as well as peak stimulated GH, which in turn stimulates IGF-I production.

SHOX-BNP and CNP-NPR2 Pathway

As discussed in the introduction, besides classical endocrine pathways, there are local mechanisms involved in growth regulation, in which hormones and their receptors play a role. One pathway which appears to be important is the pathway that is affected in patients with Leri-Weill dyschondrosteosis. A heterozygous mutation or deletion of *SHOX* or its enhancer region causes severe short stature, in the same order as seen in Turner syndrome [29]. In children previously diagnosed as idiopathic short stature, SHOX haploinsufficiency (heterozygous mutations or deletions of *SHOX* or abnormalities of the enhancer region) may be found in 2–4% [29]. It has been suggested that *BNP* is the target gene of SHOX [30]. Interestingly, a study in relatives of cases with acromesomelic dysplasia (Maroteaux type) has shown that heterozygosity for the CNP receptor (*NPR2*) may be one of the underlying causes of short stature [31]. Both observations support the hypothesis that BNP and CNP are important regulators of growth, and that defects in this pathway can cause growth disorders.

Conclusion

Growth is an extremely complex phenomenon that is regulated by a multitude of genes, part of which can be considered as belonging to the endocrine system. However, the barriers between endocrine and non-endocrine have become blurred, because most hormones and growth factors involved in this system have endocrine, paracrine and autocrine functions. Major players in growth regulation are the components of the GH-IGF-I system, thyroxine, and sex steroids. Genome-wide association studies have shown that the number of genes associated with adult height is more than 180, and the interaction between all genes and gene products are innumerable. Future studies in patients with growth disorders will undoubtedly lead to the discovery of yet unknown monogenetic growth disorders, but we believe that in the majority of short children and adults multiple genes and their interactions are involved.

References

1 Murphy VE, Smith R, Giles WB, Clifton VL: Endocrine regulation of human fetal growth: the role of the mother, placenta, and fetus. Endocr Rev 2006;27:141–169.

2 Yakar S, Liu JL, Stannard B, Butler A, Accili D, Sauer B, Leroith D: Normal growth and development in the absence of hepatic insulin-like growth factor I. Proc Natl Acad Sci USA 1999;96:7324–7329.

3 Stratikopoulos E, Szabolcs M, Dragatsis I, Klinakis A, Efstratiadis A: The hormonal action of IGF1 in postnatal mouse growth. Proc Natl Acad Sci USA 2008;105:19378–19383.

4 Wit JM, Kamp GA, Rikken B: Spontaneous growth and response to growth hormone treatment in children with growth hormone deficiency and idiopathic short stature. Pediatr Res 1996;39:295–302.

5 Alatzoglou KS, Dattani MT: Genetic forms of hypopituitarism and their manifestation in the neonatal period. Early Hum Dev 2009;85:705–712.

6 Mehta A, Gevers EF, Dattani MT: Congenital disorders of the hypothalamo-pituitary-somatotrope axis; in Brook CGD, Clayton PE, Brown RS, (eds): Brook's Clinical Pediatric Endocrinology. Oxford, Wiley-Blackwell, 2009, pp 60–105.

7 Savage MO, Attie KM, David A, Metherell LA, Clark AJ, Camacho-Hübner C: Endocrine assessment, molecular characterization and treatment of growth hormone insensitivity disorders. Nat Clin Pract Endocrinol Metab 2006;2:395–407.

8 Rosenfeld RG, Belgorosky A, Camacho-Hubner C, Savage MO, Wit JM, Hwa V: Defects in growth hormone receptor signaling. Trends Endocrinol Metab 2007;18:134–141.

9 Pugliese-Pires P, Tonelli C, Dora JM, Silva P, Czepielewski MA, Simoni G, Arnhold IJ, Jorge A: A novel STAT5b mutation causing GH insensitivity syndrome associated with hyperprolactinemia and immune dysfunction in two male siblings. Eur J Endocrinol 2010;163:349–355.

10 Padidela R, Camacho-Hübner C, Attie KM, Savage MO: Abnormal growth in Noonan syndrome: genetic and endocrine features and optimal treatment. Horm Res 2008;70:129–136.

11 Wu S, Walenkamp MJ, Lankester A, Bidlingmaier M, Wit JM, De Luca F: Growth hormone and insulin-like growth factor I insensitivity of fibroblasts isolated from a patient with an I{kappa} B{alpha} mutation. J Clin Endocrinol Metab 2010; 95:1220–1228.

12 Woods KA, Camacho-Hubner C, Savage MO, Clark AJ: Intrauterine growth retardation and postnatal growth failure associated with deletion of the insulin-like growth factor I gene. N Engl J Med 1996;335:1363–1367.

13 Walenkamp MJ, Karperien M, Pereira AM, Hilhorst-Hofstee Y, van Doorn J, Chen JW, Mohan S, Denley A, Forbes B, van Duyvenvoorde HA, van Thiel SW, Sluimers CA, Bax JJ, de Laat JA, Breuning MB, Romijn JA, Wit JM: Homozygous and heterozygous expression of a novel insulin-like growth factor-I mutation. J Clin Endocrinol Metab 2005;90:2855–2864.

14 Netchine I, Azzi S, Houang M, Seurin D, Perin L, Ricort JM, Daubas C, Legay C, Mester J, Herich R, Godeau F, Le Bouc Y: Partial primary deficiency of insulin-like growth factor (IGF)-I activity associated with IGF1 mutation demonstrates its critical role in growth and brain development. J Clin Endocrinol Metab 2009;94:3913–3921.

15 Domene HM, Hwa V, Argente J, Wit JM, Camacho-Hubner C, Jasper HG, Pozo J, van Duyvenvoorde HA, Yakar S, Fofanova-Gambetti OV, Rosenfeld RG: Human acid-labile subunit deficiency: clinical, endocrine and metabolic consequences. Horm Res 2009;72:129–141.

16 Abuzzahab MJ, Schneider A, Goddard A, Grigorescu F, Lautier C, Keller E, Kiess W, Klammt J, Kratzsch J, Osgood D, Pfäffle R, Raile K, Seidel B, Smith RJ, Chernausek SD, Intrauterine Growth Retardation (IUGR) Study Group: IGF-I receptor mutations resulting in intrauterine and postnatal growth retardation. N Engl J Med 2003;349:2211–2222.

17 Ester WA, van Duyvenvoorde HA, de Wit CC, Broekman AJ, Ruivenkamp CA, Govaerts LC, Wit JM, Hokken-Koelega AC, Losekoot M: Two short children born small for gestational age with insulin-like growth factor 1 receptor haploinsufficiency illustrate the heterogeneity of its phenotype. J Clin Endocrinol Metab 2009;94:4717–4727.

18 Murphy R, Baptista J, Holly J, Umpleby AM, Ellard S, Harries LW, Crolla J, Cundy T, Hattersley AT: Severe intrauterine growth retardation and atypical diabetes associated with a translocation breakpoint disrupting regulation of the insulin-like growth factor 2 gene. J Clin Endocrinol Metab 2008;93:4373–4380.

19 Demars J, Shmela ME, Rossignol S, Okabe J, Netchine I, Azzi S, Cabrol S, Le Caignec C, David A, Le Bouc Y, El Osta A, Gicquel C: Analysis of the IGF2/H19 imprinting control region uncovers new genetic defects, including mutations of OCT-binding sequences, in patients with 11p15 fetal growth disorders. Hum Mol Genet 2010;19:803–814.

20 Boersma B, Otten BJ, Stoelinga GB, Wit JM: Catch-up growth after prolonged hypothyroidism. Eur J Pediatr 1996;155:362–367.

21 Rivkees SA, Bode HH, Crawford JD: Long-term growth in juvenile acquired hypothyroidism: the failure to achieve normal adult stature. N Engl J Med 1988;318:599–602.

22 Burguera B, Muruais C, Penalva A, Dieguez C, Casanueva FF: Dual and selective actions of glucocorticoids upon basal and stimulated growth hormone release in man. Neuroendocrinology 1990;51: 51–58.

23 Metherell LA, Chan LF, Clark AJ: The genetics of ACTH resistance syndromes. Best Pract Res Clin Endocrinol Metab 2006;20:547–560.

24 van der Eerden BC, Karperien M, Wit JM: Systemic and local regulation of the growth plate. Endocr Rev 2003;24:782–801.

25 Oz OK, Millsaps R, Welch R, Birch J, Zerwekh JE: Expression of aromatase in the human growth plate. J Mol Endocrinol 2001;27:249–253.

26 Morishima A, Grumbach MM, Simpson ER, Fisher C, Qin K: Aromatase deficiency in male and female siblings caused by a novel mutation and the physiological role of estrogens. J Clin Endocrinol Metab 1995;80:3689–3698.

27 Ross JL, Cassorla FG, Skerda MC, Valk IM, Loriaux DL, Cutler GB: A preliminary study of the effect of estrogen dose on growth in Turner's syndrome. N Engl J Med 1983;3:1104–1106.

28 Smith EP, Boyd J, Frank GR, Takahashi H, Cohen RM, Specker B, Williams TC, Lubahn DB, Korach KS: Estrogen resistance caused by a mutation in the estrogen-receptor gene in a man. N Engl J Med 1994;331:1056–1061.

29 Rappold G, Blum WF, Shavrikova EP, Crowe BJ, Roeth R, Quigley CA, Ross JL, Niesler B: Genotypes and phenotypes in children with short stature: clinical indicators of SHOX haploinsufficiency. J Med Genet 2007;44:306–313.

30 Marchini A, Hacker B, Marttila T, Hesse V, Emons J, Weiss B, Karperien M, Rappold G: BNP is a transcriptional target of the short stature homeobox gene SHOX. Hum Mol Genet 2007;16:3081–3087.

31 Olney RC, Bukulmez H, Bartels CF, Prickett TC, Espiner EA, Potter LR, Warman ML: Heterozygous mutations in natriuretic peptide receptor-B (NPR2) are associated with short stature. J Clin Endocrinol Metab 2006;91:1229–1232.

Prof. Dr. Jan M. Wit
Department of Paediatrics, Leiden University Medical Center
PO Box 9600
NL–2300 RC Leiden (The Netherlands)
Tel. +31 71 5262824, E-Mail j.m.wit@lumc.nl

Camacho-Hübner C, Nilsson O, Sävendahl L (eds): Cartilage and Bone Development and Its Disorders.
Endocr Dev. Basel, Karger, 2011, vol 21, pp 42–51

Estrogen Signaling in Growth Plate Cartilage

Elham Karimian · Lars Sävendahl

Pediatric Endocrinology Unit, Q2:08, Department of Women's and Children's Health, Karolinska Institutet and University Hospital, Stockholm, Sweden

Abstract

It is well known that sex steroids, in particular estrogens, play an important role in longitudinal bone growth during puberty. High doses of estrogen therapy can reduce the final height of an individual, but such treatment is also associated with severe side effects. At the same time, attenuation of estrogen production by aromatase inhibitors increases adult final height, inhibiting bone turnover, which influences bone architecture and may increase the risk for vertebrae fractures. SERMs, which display either estrogenic and/or antiestrogenic effects, bind to ERs with different affinities and subsequently recruit comodulators of transcription in a tissue-specific manner.

The physiological effects of estrogens are mediated primarily by two known nuclear receptors, ERα [1, 2] and ERβ [3], each containing 6 domains (A–F) as detailed in figure 1. ERα and ERβ act as classical ligand-activated transcription factors, residing in the cytosol until binding their ligand and then being translocated into the nucleus, where the estrogen-ER complex interacts with EREs in the promoter regions of target genes. In addition, estrogens bind to subpopulations of ERα and ERβ associated with the plasma membrane, thereby rapidly activating a variety of intracellular signaling cascades.

Recently, a membrane-bound G protein-coupled estrogen receptor (GPR30) that rapidly mediates estrogen signaling was identified [4]. This receptor is expressed at high levels in the hypertrophic zone, and the expression level decreases during pubertal progression, suggesting that GPR30 is involved in modulating longitudinal bone growth [5]. The observation that estrogen treatment of mice lacking this receptor *(GPR30–/–)*, does not influence the growth plate height or femur length

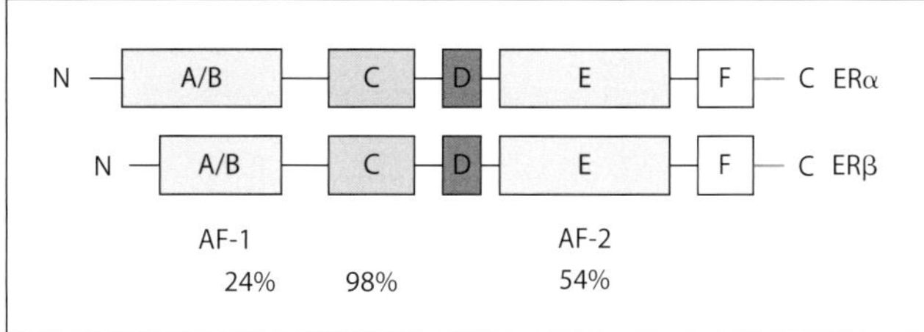

Fig. 1. Structure of the estrogen receptors. These receptors contain 6 domains (A–F). From the N to the C terminus: the A/B domain mediates ligand-independent activation (AF-1); the C domain contains the DNA-binding domain that binds to EREs in target genes; the D domain is a hinge that provides flexibility between the C and N termini. The E and F domains contain the site that binds estrogen and estrogenic compounds. The AF-1 region at the N terminus and the AF-2 region within the ligand-binding domain are involved in ligand-independent and ligand-dependent transcriptional activation, respectively. The percentages of homology between the A/B, C and E domains in these two isoforms are indicated below these domains.

[6] indicates that GPR30 is required for normal estrogenic responses in the growth plate.

Classical Mechanism of Ligand-Dependent ER Action

Ligand binding to the ER induces a conformational change that promotes ligand-receptor dimerization, and this dimeric complex is then translocated into the nucleus, where it binds to a specific ERE in the promoter regions of responsive genes and activates their transcription.

ERE-Independent Activation of Transcription

Studies have demonstrated that ERs can regulate transcription without binding directly to DNA through protein-to-protein interactions with a complex of transcription factors that have direct contact with DNA. In this way, ERs regulate the expression of a large number of genes that do not contain EREs. This mechanism, which is common among members of the nuclear receptor superfamily, is often referred to as transcriptional cross talk [7].

Ligand-Independent Effects on Transcription

Certain growth factors activate protein kinase cascades that lead to the phosphorylation and activation of nuclear ERs bound to EREs.

Nongenomic Action

Membrane E2-ER complexes activate protein kinase cascades, thereby altering the functions of various cytoplasmic proteins and/or regulating gene expression through phosphorylation and activation of transcription factors.

Endogenous Estrogen Production by Chondrocytes

Chondrocytes appear to synthesize estrogen, both in vivo and in vitro [8–10], which is in agreement with the observation that the P450 aromatase is expressed in growth plate cartilage of both humans [8] and rats [10, 11]. Moreover, local estrogen production has been reported to be essential for chondrocyte proliferation and protecting these cells from undergoing spontaneous cell death and thereby the maintenance of longitudinal bone growth [11].

Effects of Estrogen Deficiency on Bone Growth

The basic assumption that estrogen is the sex steroid primarily responsible for regulating pubertal growth in girls, while in boys this regulation is mediated primarily by androgens was challenged by Smith and his colleagues in the 1990s. These investigators described the unique case of a 28-year-old male patient referred to the surgeon for progressive genu valgum, whose radiological examination revealed unfused epiphyses, a bone age of 15 years and a lumbar spine BMD that was 3 SD below the appropriate control mean. He was 204 cm tall, had an arm span of 213 cm and he was still growing slowly during the third decade of his life. Transdermal treatment with high doses of ethinyl E2 for 6 months neither improved his total BMD nor advanced his bone age [12].

DNA analysis revealed a homozygous mutation in exon 2 of this patient's ERα gene, resulting in a substitution of thymine for cytosine. Despite his normal serum levels of androgen, this genetic estrogen resistance was associated with a delay in skeletal maturation and continuing increase in height into adulthood [12]. Histomorphometrical analysis of this patient's bones revealed that disruption of ERα actions markedly affected their mineral content and structure, but not the periosteal circumference [13].

In 1995, a male and a female sibling with a similar phenotype appearance were described, but in these cases the genetic defect was due to a homozygous mutation in exon IX of the aromatase P450 (CYP19) gene that led to high levels of androgens, but unlike the patient described by Smith et al. [12, 13], this patient had undetectable levels of serum E2 [14, 15] and responded to therapy with conjugated estrogen. These observations indicate that androgen alone is not sufficient to promote skeletal maturation and maintain bone mass and that estrogens play a pivotal role in bone mineralization in both males and females. The local expression of ERs by growth plate chondrocytes of various animal species [16, 17] indicates that estrogens exert direct effects in this context.

Estrogen Induces Fusion of the Growth Plate in Humans

Clinical cases of estrogen deficiency due to a defect in the synthesis of estrogen or function of its receptor clearly illustrate the significance of this sex hormone in regulating the pubertal growth spurt and growth plate fusion in both girls and boys [12, 14, 18]. When a child approaches the end of his or her period of growth, the growth plate thins and the rate of growth gradually declines, and finally ceases when the growth plate has vanished completely. High-dose treatment of children with E2 promotes early fusion of the growth plate via the same processes that normally occur late in puberty [19].

The mechanism by which estrogens promote epiphyseal fusion is not well understood, but there is an alternative hypothesis based on a study in rabbits. Unlike what happens in small rodents, the growth plate in rabbits fuses at the time of sexual maturation or upon estrogen treatment [20]. This hypothesis proposes that the growth plate undergoes programmed senescence, involving reductions in the rates of growth and chondrocyte proliferation, as well as the number and size of chondrocytes [20]. Moreover, growth plate fusion appears to be triggered when the proliferative capacity of the chondrocytes located there is fully exhausted.

Estrogen Treatment for Modulation of Bone Growth

When administered during adolescence, high-dose estrogen treatment has been reported to effectively reduce adult height in constitutionally tall girls [21, 22]. However, the long-term effects of such treatment are now being recognized. Today, it is known that high-dose estrogen therapy may negatively influence fertility later in life [23], increase the risk for deep vein thrombosis [24], as well as, possibly, increase the risk for breast and gynecological cancers [25]. In contrast, treatment of idiopathic short stature by blocking estrogen biosynthesis successfully delays skeletal maturation and enhances adult height without serious side effects [26]. However, a recent study in prepubertal boys treated for 6 months with an aromatase inhibitor to improve their adult final height revealed that the elevated bone resorption caused by this drug was not paralleled by an increase in bone formation [27]. Moreover, there is a strong correlation between serum levels of E2 and BMD in males [28], once again emphasizing the importance of this sex hormone for bone health in both females and males.

Lessons from Mice Lacking ERα and/or ERβ

To gain further insight into the role played by each individual ER, ERKO, BERKO or DERKO mice strains have been generated [29–31]. ERKO mice generated in the laboratory of Dr. Smithies [32–37] express a truncated form of ERα produced by alternative splicing [38], whereas BERKO mice generated in Dr. Smithies' laboratory express no ERβ at all. An ERKO mouse strain generated in the laboratory of Dr. Chambon [39, 40] is considered to be ERα-null, with no ER activity, whereas BERKO mice from the same group express isoforms of ERβ.

The femur length of adult or elderly female ERKO mice has been reported to be either normal [39, 40] or reduced [33, 41]. On the other hand, male ERKO mice show decreased bone growth, both as adults [35] and upon aging [41]. In male BERKO mice bone growth is unaffected throughout development [35–37, 39], while in adult female BERKO mice bone length is increased [32–33, 37]. Interestingly, in male DERKO mice bone growth is decreased to the same extent as in the ERKO strain [35], while in females, DERKO animals have longer bones than ERKO [32–33]. Altogether, these observations suggest that ERβ has a negative impact on longitudinal bone growth. The difference between the phenotype of the unique clinical case with a mutated ERα and the knockout mouse models might reflect species differences with regard to the functions of ER isoforms. Moreover, the diverse phenotypes of male and female ER-knockout mice indicate the existence of sex-related differences in ER functions.

Direct Effects of Estrogens on Chondrocytes

Indeed, the expression of ERα [42], ERβ [16] and GPR30 [5] by human epiphyseal chondrocytes supports direct actions of estrogens on these cells. However, at physiological levels E2 does not influence cell proliferation and viability, synthesis of type X collagen, alkaline phosphatase activity, or matrix calcification in primary cultures of resting, proliferating, and prehypertrophic chondrocytes derived from the bovine fetal epiphyseal growth plate [43]. The effect of estrogens on longitudinal bone growth in vivo, but not in vitro suggests the presence of a cofactor in vivo which is lacking in cultures or, alternatively, that local production of estrogen in cultures masks the effects of exogenous estrogens [11].

Selective Estrogen Receptor Modulators

Thanks to their selective effects, certain SERMs can be used to prevent or treat diseases caused by estrogen deficiency, such as osteoporosis, without most of the undesirable side effects of estrogens. Conversely, other SERMs act as selective estrogen antagonists, and can therefore be used to prevent or treat diseases, such as breast cancer, in which estrogen activity in a particular tissue is undesirable.

Thus, unlike estrogens, which are all agonists, and antiestrogens, which are all antagonists, SERMs include a diversity of compounds that can act as either ER agonists or antagonists in a tissue-specific manner [44]. This pharmacological specificity allows dissociation of desirable estrogenic effects on the bone from undesirable stimulatory effects on the breast and endometrium. These compounds all lack the steroid structure of estrogens, but possess a tertiary structure that allows them to bind to the ERs. Most, but probably not all of their agonistic and antagonistic activities on target tissues for estrogens can be explained by three major interacting factors: differences in the levels of ERα and ERβ expression, differences in the conformational ER changes that occur upon ligand binding and differences in the expression of coregulator proteins (coactivators or corepressors) [45].

PhytoSERMs are plant products that have been shown to exert similar actions as synthetic SERMs. Like other SERMs, these compounds act on the ERs in a selective manner, either as agonists or antagonists, thereby offering the possibility of selectively stimulating or inhibiting estrogen-like responses in different tissues. At present, two well-characterized classes of chemical SERMs have been approved for clinical use, whereas phytoSERMs are still under investigation.

Tamoxifen: A First-Generation SERM

Initially developed as an oral contraceptive, tamoxifen was actually found to induce ovulation in sub-fertile women and subsequently marketed for this purpose instead. In the early 1970s, following promising preliminary results in postmenopausal patients with breast cancer [46], this drug was reclassified as an anticancer agent and is now the most widely used adjuvant therapy in the treatment of breast cancer.

Although experience of its use in children has been limited, tamoxifen has been tested as a treatment for pubertal gynecomastia in adolescent boys [47, 48] and precocious puberty in patients with McCune-Albright syndrome [49]. In these studies, longitudinal growth was either unaffected or diminished following months of treatment [47–49]. Differences in skeletal growth in response to tamoxifen treatment might reflect the use of heterogeneous groups of patients of different ages and stages of sexual maturation. In gonadectomized male and female rats, tamoxifen causes a narrowing of the growth plate [50, 51]. Furthermore, in intact young male rats tamoxifen treatment inhibits longitudinal bone growth, an effect associated with elevated chondrocyte apoptosis, narrowing of the tibial growth plate and a reduction in serum levels of IGF-I [52]. In addition, tamoxifen induced persistent reduction in cortical bone size as a result of attenuated periosteal and endosteal growth of the cortical bone [52]. These findings suggest that if administered to growing children, tamoxifen may diminish their growth potential as well as increase their risk for bone fractures.

Raloxifene: A Second-Generation SERM

Raloxifene acts as an estrogen agonist with regard to bone density and as an estrogen antagonist in breast and uterine tissues [53], thus exerting beneficial effects on postmenopausal osteoporosis [44]. In rats, this compound inhibits longitudinal bone growth [54], while in ovariectomized rabbits it acts as an estrogen agonist on the growth plate accelerating chondrocyte senescence and thereby hastening epiphyseal fusion [55]. However, Zirrilli et al. [15] recently reported that, unlike the effect in rats and rabbits, raloxifene does not accelerate epiphyseal fusion, but does enhance BMD and circulating levels of gonadotropins in aromatase-deficient humans. This lack of efficacy of raloxifene on growth plate ossification and mineralization in aromatase-deficient humans may reflect either the low serum concentrations of the drug or species differences in the response to this drug.

Resveratrol: A phytoSERM

The existence of phytoestrogens (plant compounds with estrogenic activity) has been known for more than 75 years [56]. Despite their possible role as endocrine disrupters, in the past few decades phytoestrogens have become widely regarded as beneficial to human health, because of observations that populations whose diets contain high levels of such compounds have lower rates of certain estrogen-mediated conditions, such as cardiac disease, breast cancer, osteoporosis, and menopausal symptoms [57].

Trans-resveratrol, a polyphenolic compound, is produced in response to stress, injury and infection by a variety of plants, including peanuts, berries, red grapes, where it is located in the skin, and the Asian cane *Polygonum cuspidatum*. Its structural similarity to the potent synthetic estrogen diethylstilbestrol suggested that trans-resveratrol might be estrogenic, and, indeed, Gehm et al. [58] demonstrated that this compound can compete with labeled E2 for receptor binding, activate the expression of estrogen-regulated genes, and stimulate the growth of estrogen-dependent breast cancer cells. However, the binding affinity to the ER is rather low [59].

Resveratrol competes with E2 for binding to ER in an extract from MCF-7 human breast cancer cells with an IC_{50} value of approximately 10 μM [58] and, furthermore, binds to rat uterine ER with an IC_{50} value of 100 μM [60].

Interestingly, it has been reported that resveratrol is able to show antiestrogenic effects via inhibition of the aromatase P450, CYP19, enzyme in breast cancer cells in vitro [61]. This compound inhibited aromatase activity with an IC_{50} value of 25 μM [61].

However, it should be pointed out that when administered orally, resveratrol has low bioavailability [62–64] and, therefore, relatively high doses must be administered in order to achieve such serum concentrations. At present, pharmacological doses of resveratrol should be avoided since this compound can cause life-threatening symptoms, including kidney damage [64], at least in rats.

In growing rats, resveratrol exhibits little or no agonistic estrogen influence on reproductive and nonreproductive tissues that are targets for estrogens and may, indeed, act as an estrogen antagonist [65]. At the same time, it is well known that resveratrol displays numerous mechanisms of biological action, targeting a great number of pathways not involving estrogen receptors [66].

Conclusion

Data in experimental models as well as clinical observations in patients with de novo mutations have clarified the importance of estrogen actions for the local regulation of growth plate cartilage. Improved knowledge regarding the mechanisms of these actions could lead to new treatment strategies for children with diseases affecting longitudinal bone growth.

References

1 Green S, Walter P, Greene G, et al: Cloning of the human oestrogen receptor cDNA. J Steroid Biochem 1986;24:77–83.

2 Greene GL, Gilna P, Waterfield M, et al: Sequence and expression of human estrogen receptor complementary DNA. Science 1986;231:1150–1154.

3 Kuiper GG, Enmark E, Pelto-Huikko M, et al: Cloning of a novel receptor expressed in rat prostate and ovary. Proc Natl Acad Sci USA 1996;93:5925–5930.

4 Revankar CM, Cimino DF, Sklar LA, et al: A transmembrane intracellular estrogen receptor mediates rapid cell signaling. Science 2005;307:1625–1630.

5 Chagin AS, Sävendahl L: GPR30 estrogen receptor expression in the growth plate declines as puberty progresses. J Clin Endocrinol Metab 2007;92:4873–4877.

6 Windahl SH, Andersson N, Chagin AS, et al: The role of the G protein-coupled receptor GPR30 in the effects of estrogen in ovariectomized mice. Am J Physiol Endocrinol Metab 2009;296:E490—E496.

7 Gottlicher M, Heck S, Herrlich P: Transcriptional cross-talk, the second mode of steroid hormone receptor action. J Mol Med 1998;76:480–489.

8 Oz OK, Millsaps R, Welch R, et al: Expression of aromatase in the human growth plate. J Mol Endocrinol 2001;27:249–253.

9 Sylvia VL, Gay I, Hardin R, et al: Rat costochondral chondrocytes produce 17beta-estradiol and regulate its production by 1alpha,25(OH)(2)D(3). Bone 2002;30:57–63.

10 van der Eerden BC, Van De Ven J, Lowik CW, et al: Sex steroid metabolism in the tibial growth plate of the rat. Endocrinology 2002;143:4048–4055.

11 Chagin AS, Chrysis D, Takigawa M, et al: Locally produced estrogen promotes fetal rat metatarsal bone growth; an effect mediated through increased chondrocyte proliferation and decreased apoptosis. J Endocrinol 2006;188:193–203.

12 Smith EP, Boyd J, Frank GR, et al: Estrogen resistance caused by a mutation in the estrogen-receptor gene in a man. N Engl J Med 1994;331:1056–1061.

13 Smith EP, Specker B, Bachrach BE, et al: Impact on bone of an estrogen receptor-alpha gene loss of function mutation. J Clin Endocrinol Metab 2008;93:3088–3096.

14 Morishima A, Grumbach MM, Simpson ER, et al: Aromatase deficiency in male and female siblings caused by a novel mutation and the physiological role of estrogens. J Clin Endocrinol Metab 1995;80:3689–3698.

15 Zirilli L, Maffei L, Meunier PJ, et al: The effects of long-term raloxifene and estradiol treatments on bone in a patient with congenital aromatase deficiency. Bone 2009;45:827–832.

16 Nilsson LO, Boman A, Sävendahl L, et al: Demonstration of estrogen receptor-beta immunoreactivity in human growth plate cartilage. J Clin Endocrinol Metab 1999;84:370–373.

17 Nilsson O, Abad V, Chrysis D, et al: Estrogen receptor-alpha and -beta are expressed throughout postnatal development in the rat and rabbit growth plate. J Endocrinol 2002;173:407–414.

18 Carani C, Qin K, Simoni M, et al: Effect of testosterone and estradiol in a man with aromatase deficiency. N Engl J Med 1997;337:91–95.

19 Drop SL, De Waal WJ, De Muinck SM: Keizer-Schrama, Sex steroid treatment of constitutionally tall stature. Endocr Rev 1998;19:540–558.

20 Weise M, De-Levi S, Barnes KM, et al: Effects of estrogen on growth plate senescence and epiphyseal fusion. Proc Natl Acad Sci USA 2001;98:6871–6876.

21 Venn A, Hosmer T, Hosmer D, et al: Oestrogen treatment for tall stature in girls: estimating the effect on height and the error in height prediction. Clin Endocrinol (Oxf) 2008;68:926–929.

22 Goldzieher MA: Treatment of excessive growth in the adolescent female. J Clin Endocrinol Metab 1956;16:249–252.

23 Hendriks AEJ, Laven JSE, Valkenburg O, et al: Fertility and ovarian function in high-dose estrogen-treated tall women. J Clin Endocrinol Metab 2011;96:1098–1105.

24 Weimann E, Brack C: Severe thrombosis during treatment with ethinylestradiol for tall stature. Horm Res 1996;45:261–263.

25 Genazzani AR, Gadducci A, Gambacciani M: Controversial issues in climacteric medicine II. Hormone replacement therapy and cancer. Maturitas 2001;40:117–130.

26 Hero M, Norjavaara E, Dunkel L: Inhibition of estrogen biosynthesis with a potent aromatase inhibitor increases predicted adult height in boys with idiopathic short stature: a randomized controlled trial. J Clin Endocrinol Metab 2005;90:6396–6402.

27 Hero M, Mäkitie O, Kröger H, et al: Impact of aromatase inhibitor therapy on bone turnover, cortical bone growth and vertebral morphology in pre- and peripubertal boys with idiopathic short stature. Horm Res 2009;71:290–297.

28 Slemenda CW, Longcope C, Zhou L, et al: Sex steroids and bone mass in older men. Positive associations with serum estrogens and negative associations with androgens. J Clin Invest 1997;100:1755–1759.

29 Dupont S, Krust A, Gansmuller A, et al: Effect of single and compound knockouts of estrogen receptors alpha (ERalpha) and beta (ERbeta) on mouse reproductive phenotypes. Development 2000;127: 4277–4291.

30 Krege JH, Hodgin JB, Couse JF, et al: Generation and reproductive phenotypes of mice lacking estrogen receptor beta. Proc Natl Acad Sci USA 1998;95: 15677–15682.

31 Lubahn DB, Moyer JS, Golding TS, et al: Alteration of reproductive function but not prenatal sexual development after insertional disruption of the mouse estrogen receptor gene. Proc Natl Acad Sci USA 1993;90:11162–11166.

32 Chagin AS, Lindberg MK, Andersson N, et al: Estrogen receptor-beta inhibits skeletal growth and has the capacity to mediate growth plate fusion in female mice. J Bone Miner Res 2004;19:72–77.

33 Lindberg MK, Alatalo SL, Halleen JM, et al: Estrogen receptor specificity in the regulation of the skeleton in female mice. J Endocrinol 2001;171:229–236.

34 Vidal O, Lindberg M, Sävendahl L, et al: Disproportional body growth in female estrogen receptor-alpha-inactivated mice. Biochem Biophys Res Commun 1999;265:569–571.

35 Vidal O, Lindberg MK, Hollberg K, et al: Estrogen receptor specificity in the regulation of skeletal growth and maturation in male mice. Proc Natl Acad Sci USA 2000;97:5474–5479.

36 Windahl SH, Hollberg K, Vidal O, et al: Female estrogen receptor beta-/- mice are partially protected against age-related trabecular bone loss. J Bone Miner Res 2001;16:1388–1398.

37 Windahl SH, Vidal O, Andersson G, et al: Increased cortical bone mineral content but unchanged trabecular bone mineral density in female ERbeta–/– mice. J Clin Invest 1999;104:895–901.

38 Pendaries C, Darblade B, Rochaix P, et al: The AF-1 activation-function of ERalpha may be dispensable to mediate the effect of estradiol on endothelial NO production in mice. Proc Natl Acad Sci USA 2002;99:2205–2210.

39 Sims NA, Dupont S, Krust A, et al: Deletion of estrogen receptors reveals a regulatory role for estrogen receptors-beta in bone remodeling in females but not in males. Bone 2002;30:18–25.

40 Tozum TF, Oppenlander ME, Koh-Paige AJ, et al: Effects of sex steroid receptor specificity in the regulation of skeletal metabolism. Calcif Tissue Int 2004;75:60–70.

41 Parikka V, Peng Z, Hentunen T, et al: Estrogen responsiveness of bone formation in vitro and altered bone phenotype in aged estrogen receptor-alpha-deficient male and female mice. Eur J Endocrinol 2005;152:301–314.

42 Kusec V, Virdi AS, Prince R, Triffitt JT: Localization of estrogen receptor-alpha in human and rabbit skeletal tissues. J Clin Endocrinol Metab 1998;83: 2421–2428.

43 Rodd C, Jourdain N, Alini M: Action of estradiol on epiphyseal growth plate chondrocytes. Calcif Tissue Int 2004;75:214–224.

44 Cho CH, Nuttall ME: Therapeutic potential of oestrogen receptor ligands in development for osteoporosis. Expert Opin Emerg Drugs 2001;6:137–154.

45 Riggs BL, Hartmann LC: Selective estrogen-receptor modulators – mechanisms of action and application to clinical practice. N Engl J Med 2003;348: 618–629.

46 Cole MP, Jones CT, Todd ID: A new anti-oestrogenic agent in late breast cancer. An early clinical appraisal of ICI46474. Br J Cancer 1971;25:270–275.

47 Derman O, Kanbur NO, Kutluk T: Tamoxifen treatment for pubertal gynecomastia. Int J Adolesc Med Health 2003;15:359–363.
48 Lawrence SE, Faught KA, Vethamuthu J, Lawson ML: Beneficial effects of raloxifene and tamoxifen in the treatment of pubertal gynecomastia. J Pediatr 2004;145:71–76.
49 Eugster EA, Rubin SD, Reiter EO, et al: Tamoxifen treatment for precocious puberty in McCune-Albright syndrome: a multicenter trial. J Pediatr 2003;143:60–66.
50 Fitts JM, Klein RM, Powers CA: Comparison of tamoxifen and testosterone propionate in male rats: differential prevention of orchidectomy effects on sex organs, bone mass, growth, and the growth hormone-IGF-I axis. J Androl 2004;25:523–534.
51 Li X, Takahashi M, Kushida K, et al: The effect of tamoxifen on bone metabolism and skeletal growth is different in ovariectomized and intact rats. Calcif Tissue Int 1996;59:271–276.
52 Karimian E, Chagin AS, Gjerde J, et al: Tamoxifen impairs both longitudinal and cortical bone growth in young male rats. J Bone Miner Res 2008;23:1267–1277.
53 Barrett-Connor E: Raloxifene: risks and benefits. Ann N Y Acad Sci 2001;949:295–303.
54 Evans G, Bryant HU, Magee D, et al: The effects of raloxifene on tibia histomorphometry in ovariectomized rats. Endocrinology 1994;134:2283–2288.
55 Nilsson O, Falk J, Ritzén EM, et al: Raloxifene acts as an estrogen agonist on the rabbit growth plate. Endocrinology 2003;144:1481–1485.
56 Bradbury RB, White DE: Estrogens and related substances in plants. Vitam Horm 1954;12:207–233.
57 Bharat B, Aggarwal SS: Resveratrol in Health and Disease. London, Taylor & Francis, 2006.
58 Gehm BD, McAndrews JM, Chien PY, Jameson JL: Resveratrol, a polyphenolic compound found in grapes and wine, is an agonist for the estrogen receptor. Proc Natl Acad Sci USA 1997;94:14138–14143.
59 Bowers JL, Tyulmenkov VV, Jernigan SC, Klinge CM: Resveratrol acts as a mixed agonist/antagonist for estrogen receptors alpha and beta. Endocrinology 2000;141:3657–3667.
60 Ashby J, Tinwell H, Pennie W, et al: Partial and weak oestrogenicity of the red wine constituent resveratrol: consideration of its superagonist activity in MCF-7 cells and its suggested cardiovascular protective effects. J Appl Toxicol 1999;19:39–45.
61 Wang Y, Lee KW, Chan FL, et al: The red wine polyphenol resveratrol displays bilevel inhibition on aromatase in breast cancer cells. Toxicol Sci 2006;92:71–77.
62 Baur JA, Sinclair DA: Therapeutic potential of resveratrol: the in vivo evidence. Nat Rev Drug Discov 2006:5:493–506.
63 Bhat KP, Lantvit D, Christov K, et al: Estrogenic and antiestrogenic properties of resveratrol in mammary tumor models. Cancer Res 2001;61:7456–7463.
64 Crowell JA, Korytko PJ, Morrissey RL, et al: Resveratrol-associated renal toxicity. Toxicol Sci 2004;82:614–619.
65 Turner RT, Evans GL, Zhang M, et al: Is resveratrol an estrogen agonist in growing rats? Endocrinology 1999;140:50–54.
66 Shakibaei M, Harikumar KB, Aggarwal BB: Resveratrol addiction: to die or not to die. Mol Nutr Food Res 2009;53:115–128.

Prof. Lars Sävendahl
Pediatric Endocrinology Unit, Q2:08, Department of Women's and Children's Health
Karolinska Institutet and University Hospital
SE–171 76 Stockholm (Sweden)
Tel. +46 8 5177 2369, E-Mail lars.savendahl@ki.se

Camacho-Hübner C, Nilsson O, Sävendahl L (eds): Cartilage and Bone Development and Its Disorders.
Endocr Dev. Basel, Karger, 2011, vol 21, pp 52–66

Methods to Study Cartilage and Bone Development

Anenisia C. Andrade[a] · Dionisios Chrysis[b] · Laura Audi[c] · Ola Nilsson[a]

[a]Department of Women's and Children's Health, Karolinska Institutet, Stockholm, Sweden; [b]Division of Endocrinology, Department of Paediatrics, Medical School, University of Patras, Patras, Greece; [c]Paediatric Endocrinology Research Unit, Research Institute, Department of Paediatrics, Hospital Vall d'Hebron, Autonomous University, Centre for Biomedical Research Network on Rare Diseases, Instituto de Salud Carlos III, Barcelona, Spain

Abstract

In humans, the study of linear growth at the level of growth plate is limited to the use of mainly noninvasive methods. The use of in vitro studies and diverse animal models are alternative applied methods to unravel the underlying mechanisms of endochondral ossification and bone remodeling. In this chapter, we will outline important techniques to study molecular interactions and the regulation of gene expression in chondrocytes as well as bone cells. Microdissection of growth plate provides a powerful approach to study gene expression of individual zones and temporal senescence of growth plate cartilage by using microarray and real-time PCR analysis. IHC gives valuable information about the distribution of proteins of interest throughout distinct layers of the growth plate. The TUNEL assay has been successfully applied to study apoptosis in chondrocytes. In addition, organ (metatarsal) culture, primary and cell line cultures have been widely used to explore the regulation of chondrocyte differentiation under varying experimental conditions. Ultimately, these methods are essential to give new insights into the search for new diagnostic and therapeutic approaches for growth and various metabolic bone disorders.

In humans, the study of linear growth at the level of growth plate is limited to the use of mainly noninvasive methods. Although studies of human skeletal development are possible in the embryo and the fetus, providing useful data on gene expression and protein synthesis at this early stage of bone development [1], the use of in vitro studies and diversified animal models are alternative methods applied to unravel the underlying mechanisms of endochondral ossification and bone remodeling. Recently, advances in molecular biology have allowed for genetic manipulation and generation of animal models resulting in new understanding of specific genes during growth and development [2].

Using a panel of different techniques on growth plates, metatarsal culture, and cell culture models, complex molecular interactions and the regulation of gene expression may be studied in bone cells and chondrocytes. Primary cells derived from cartilage and bone of human and other species have been successfully cultured [3, 4]. While primary cells resemble in vivo conditions more closely, chondrocytic cell lines and cells derived from osteoblastic tumors are also widely used [5]. Ultimately, these methods are essential to give new insights into the search for novel diagnostic and therapeutic approaches for growth and metabolic bone disorders.

Considering all these perspectives, we outline important and available methodologies to further explore gene expression, signaling and interaction of molecular pathways that regulate endochondral ossification. Specifically, in this chapter we discuss in some detail the methods used in growth plate microdissection, IHC, culture of metatarsals, chondrocytic cell lines and primary human fetal chondrocytes. We also highlight how these tools may be used to study cartilage and bone development.

Growth Plate Microdissection and Gene Expression

Manual microdissection is a reliable and accurate technique that allows the study of distinct zones of growth plate cartilage from single animals [6]. This technique, like laser-capture microdissection, allows visual inspection of growth plate cartilage and hence, the dissection of individual zones of growth plate. Unlike laser-capture microdissection, manual microdissection does not require expensive equipment, avoids overheating and possible tissue damage that may result from the laser, and permits the use of thicker sections, thus decreasing the required number of dissections.

The technique is applicable to growth plate tissue collected from any mammalian species, including human. In our experience, as it is the most inexpensive and readily available laboratory animal, the rodent has been most extensively used for postnatal bone growth studies [7, 8]. Furthermore, rodents have well-annotated genomes, allowing for the use of microarray analysis and other techniques applicable to genomic studies. Unlike in humans, growth plates do not fuse in rodents, but cell proliferation reaches a very low rate, near zero [9]. In addition, the shorter lifespan of these animals makes this model useful to study temporal changes in growth plate that includes growth deceleration.

Growth plate cartilage contains distinct zones that represent discrete stages of chondrocyte differentiation, which can be distinguished by histological landmarks (fig. 1). In order to dissect zones of interest, we collect proximal tibial growth plates of young animals, e.g. 7-day-old rodents. At this age, the height of the growth plate is relatively big, and the characteristic histology is easy to appreciate. In addition, enough material is commonly obtained from individual zones from single animals to extract RNA and perform further analysis. Frozen longitudinal sections (40–60 μm) of proximal tibial growth plates are mounted on Superfrost Plus slides (Fisher

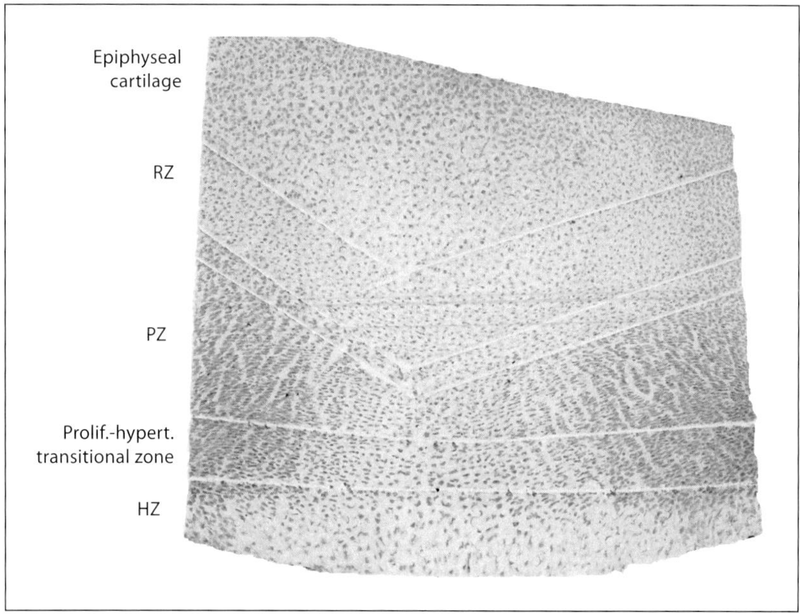

Fig. 1. Photomicrograph of a frozen longitudinal section (60 μm) from a proximal tibial growth plate from 7-day-old rats. The section has been cut with a blade to separate the growth plate into epiphyseal cartilage, RZ, PZ, proliferative-hypertrophic transitional zone, and HZ. To minimize cross-contamination between the RZ and the PZ, we discarded a segment of cartilage containing the transition area between RZ and PZ. From Nilsson et al. [6], with permission.

Scientific, Chicago, Ill., USA) and stored at –80°C. The following paragraphs describe the procedures where approximately 50 up to 200 ng of intact total RNA may be extracted from individual growth plate zones from a single animal. In this section, growth plate structure, identification of zone boundaries, and stepwise details of the procedure are addressed.

Dissection of Epiphyseal Growth Plates and Tissue Processing

Rats (Sprague-Dawley) or mice (C57BL/6) are sacrificed by CO_2 inhalation, or decapitation of younger animals. Proximal tibial epiphyses are rapidly excised, trimmed of cortical bone and placed in opposite corners of cryomolds (15 × 15 mm) placed on dry ice. Cortical bone is trimmed off the medial face of the bone in order to facilitate cryosectioning of tissue and also to provide steady placement of the epiphysis during embedding in optimum cutting temperature compound (Sakur Finetek, Torrance, Calif., USA). The tissue specimens are stored at –80°C for subsequent processing. The entire tissue collecting process should be performed in a clean environment, and completed within 10 min for each animal in order to minimize RNA degradation.

Sample Sectioning

The sectioning of samples is made in a regular cryostat on Superfrost plus slides. The ideal sample thickness should be between 40 and 60 μm. Precautions to minimize RNA degradation of growth plate sample should be made, such as cleaning the working environment with RNase solution, as well as working as fast as possible.

The methodology is as follows: (1) place a metal plate on dry ice and allow sufficient time (about 5 min) to cool down; (2) then, make the sections and place them on Superfrost plus slides, one section per slide. Immediately (within 5 s) put the slide on the pre-cooled metal surface. Make sure that the metal surface is cold enough to freeze the section within 10 s. Note that RNA degrades rapidly at temperature above 0°C and every effort to shorten this time should therefore be undertaken. Approximately 25 slides from each block can be obtained, starting from the center of the sample. After sectioning, quickly transfer the slides to a pre-cooled slide box without removing the slides from the box filled with dry ice. Store the slide box at –80°C.

Pretreatment of Slides (Fixation and Staining)

Before the start of microdissection, thaw slides completely for approximately 30 s, and immediately place in 70% ethanol for 1 min. Then, fix the slides and stain by 1-min incubations in the following solutions and in the following order: 100% methanol, 95% ethanol, and eosin (0.2% eosin, 0.5% acetic acid, 75% ethanol). The slides are subsequently dehydrated in graded ethanol bath (1 min each): 70% ethanol, 100% ethanol, 100% ethanol, and then placed in xylene (100%).

Microdissection of Growth Plate

Using an inverted microscope, razor blades, and hypodermic needles, growth plate sections are carefully separated under a xylene droplet based on histological landmarks of distinct zones (fig. 1). In the epiphysis, before the secondary ossification center develops, single chondrocytes are round and randomly oriented. The RZ contains small and rounded chondrocytes that are isolated or distributed in pairs. In the PZ, chondrocytes are flat, and arranged in columns oriented along the long axis of the bone. The transitional zone contains a mixed population of proliferative and hypertrophic chondrocytes with increased cytoplasmic volume. In the HZ, chondrocytes are distinguished from PZ chondrocytes by their apparent larger size and smaller nucleus. In addition, perichondrium and metaphyseal bone may be collected from the same sections. Metaphyseal bone can be obtained from a region of trabecular bone

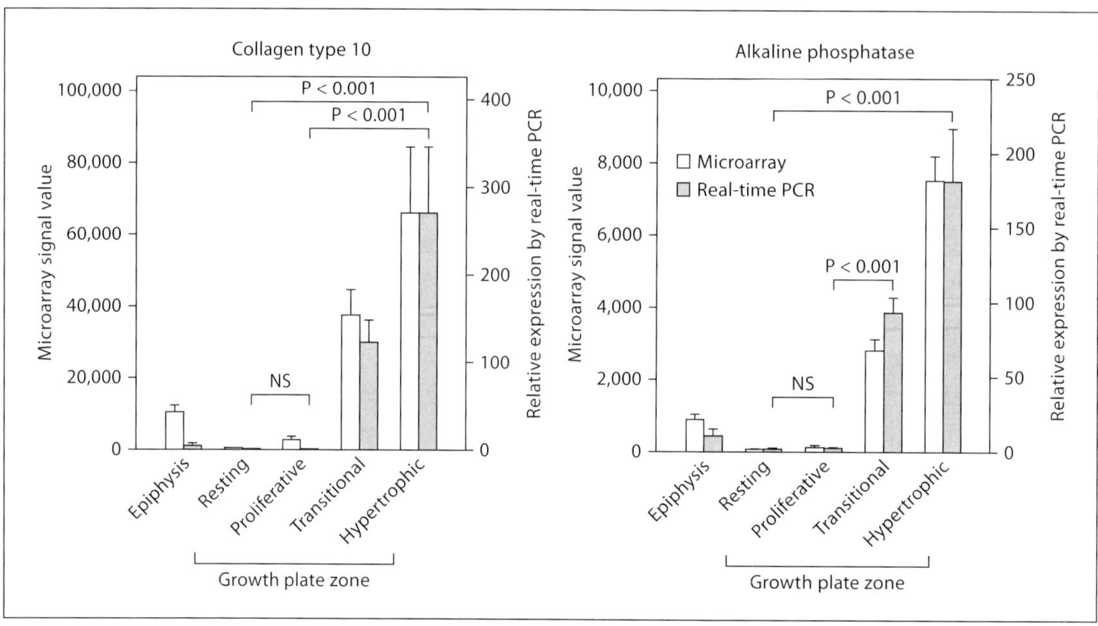

Fig. 2. Validation of growth plate microdissection. Relative expression of type X collagen and alkaline phosphatase mRNA in microdissected growth plate cartilage was determined using microarray analysis (n = 5) and real-time PCR (n = 7). Microarray signal values were background corrected and normalized. Relative expression values generated by real-time PCR were normalized to 18S rRNA. NS = Not significant. From Nilsson et al. [6], with permission.

beginning approximately 30–40 µm distal to the HZ. Cortical bone may also be collected from the slides. In order to minimize cross-contamination, narrow segments of tissue between each zone should be discarded. Even with every precaution taken, some low-grade cross-contamination may still occur. Any small amount of cross-contamination would tend to decrease differences in mRNA levels between adjacent zones. Therefore, the actual differences in mRNA expression between adjacent zones and tissues may be even greater than the ones that have been observed using this technique. Once the slides are stained and placed in xylene, the microdissection must be done in the next few hours and collected samples kept on ice. Pieces of microdissected cartilage are placed in 100 µl of 'solution C', a solution consisting of 4 M guanidine, thiocyanate, 25 mM sodium citrate, pH 7.0, and 0.1 M β-mercaptoethanol (Sigma-Aldrich, St. Louis, Mo., USA).

The accuracy of the microdissection technique was previously validated by the assessment of established markers for HZ, using microarray and real-time PCR. Type X collagen and alkaline phosphatase mRNA were detected at approximately 250- and 100-fold higher levels in HZ compared to PZ, respectively, suggesting that manual microdissection provides an accurate separation of these zones (fig. 2) [6].

Total RNA Extraction

For each zone of growth plate, dissections from both proximal tibias of one animal (18–25 sections) are pooled in individual Eppendorf tubes containing 100 μl of 'solution C'. RNA isolation is performed as previously described [10], except that one tenth of every volume and higher concentration of guanidine thiocyanate (4 M) is used in the protocol for microdissected growth plate. The RNA pellet was resuspended in diethylpyrocarbonate-treated water, usually 5 μl for microarray and 10 μl for cDNA synthesis. Digestion of cartilage by proteinase K at the beginning of the protocol and the 'clean-up' with 8 M lithium chloride in the end of the protocol are essential procedures to produce intact RNA with a yield sufficient for microarray and real-time PCR analysis. Evaluation of integrity and concentration of RNA is assessed by using RNA Pico Chips in a Bioanalyzer 2100 (Agilent Biotechnologies, Inc., Palo Alto, Calif., USA), according to manufacturer's instructions. For each animal, approximately 50–200 ng of total RNA is extracted from individual zones of the growth plate, as well as from the metaphyseal bone. To remove any residual genomic DNA from the purified total RNA, DNase treatment may be performed using DNA-free (Applied Biosystems; Foster City, Calif., USA) according to manufacturer's instruction. DNase treatment decreases the detection of genomic DNA, especially in cases where the design of primers cannot be mRNA specific where genes contain only one single exon [11].

Applications of Growth Plate Microdissection

The most important application of manual microdissection is the combination of microarray and real-time PCR analysis, providing a powerful quantitative approach to study mRNA expression in growth plate cartilage. A genome-wide analysis of growth plate cartilage allows the identification of new markers and novel signaling pathways that play an important role not only in the distinct stages of chondrocyte differentiation in individual zones, but also in the temporal regulation of chondrocyte proliferation and differentiation during postnatal chondrogenesis [8].

In vitro Methods in Growth Plate Research

Immunohistochemistry

IHC is the method by which proteins of interest are detected on tissue sections in individual cells. Briefly, the principle of the method is the following. Tissue sections fixed on slides are incubated with antibody against the protein of interest (primary antibody). Then, they are incubated with an antibody against the immunoglobulin of the species in which the primary antibody was raised (secondary antibody). The secondary antibody is linked to a system producing color.

The chondrocytes of the three different layers forming the growth plate (resting, proliferative, hypertrophic) have different functions, may produce different proteins, and they can be influenced by different factors. Thus, IHC can give valuable information about the distribution of a certain protein throughout the three layers of the growth plate, if it is located in the nucleus, cytoplasm or both. As an example, a protein can be expressed in only one layer, in two, or only at the end of a layer like the terminal hypertrophic chondrocytes. Developmental changes of a protein can also be examined by IHC, giving indirect information about the role or importance of the protein at certain developmental stages. In addition, we can study whether various experimental conditions during in vivo experiments can affect proteins of interest at the growth plate. As an example, dexamethasone treatment decreases dramatically the antiapoptotic protein Bcl-2 in the growth plate [12].

Technical Issues

For IHC, bones are usually decalcified, then formalin fixed, and finally paraffin embedded. Fixation with formalin provides better morphology of the tissue compared to frozen tissues. On the other hand, formaldehyde-based fixatives can cross-link proteins in tissues. This can mask antigen epitopes of the protein, making them inaccessible to the specific antibodies, resulting in false-negative results. Protein cross-linking can be removed by antigen retrieval which can be performed by either enzyme digestion or heating the tissues in certain solutions. One of the well-established methods of antigen retrieval is heating the tissues in citric acid (0.01 M, pH = 6.0) [13]. Antigen retrieval enhances the sensitivity of the immunostaining, and it is possible to decrease the concentration of the primary antibody and thereby diminish the risk for nonspecific staining. Antigen retrieval by heating may also cause some problems with the morphology of the growth plate. Tissues are often detached from the slides or misfolded maybe because their consistency is so different from the adjacent bone, and they become easily detached when boiled. We have found that by keeping the temperature during the procedure of antigen retrieval at 95–98°C without boiling, we can decrease the above-mentioned problems in sections from growth plates.

For the development of the color, there are different enzymatic systems, the most important being the peroxidase, alkaline phosphatase, and glucose oxidase systems. The peroxidase enzymatic system is the most commonly used since it gives the opportunity for different soluble or insoluble colored products depending on the substrate. DAB is the most commonly used substrate since it is permanent, sensitive and gives a dense stain. Although the final step of IHC, the counter stain, is simple, it is important for the quality of the experiment. If the protein of interest has a nuclear localization, then we use a cytoplasmatic stain and vice versa. Finally, the color of the counter stain has to be compatible with the color of the substrate enzyme. When using DAB, which gives brown dense color, the methyl green and the Alcian blue stains for the growth plate are good choices since they stain lightly only the collagen.

We have used IHC in the growth plate with stable and reliable results. For the detailed protocol, see Chrysis et al. [14]. We have found that several washing steps (up to 10) for short time contribute to less specific staining rather than the conventional 3 washings for long time [14].

Specificity

One of the most important issues in IHC is the specificity of the antibodies. In order to minimize problems with specificity before any experiment, one should consider the following actions whenever possible. (1) It is always better to use an antibody that has been used before with confirmed specificity. (2) A polyclonal antibody recognizes more epitopes of an antigen, and therefore it is possible to recognize the antigen of interest compared to a monoclonal which recognizes just one epitope. On the other hand, a monoclonal antibody can be more specific than a polyclonal antibody. (3) It is very important to include positive and negative controls. A tissue that contains cells that express and others that do not express the protein of interest is the ideal control tissue. (4) Preabsorption of the primary antibody with the appropriate antigen, when this is available, should abolish the staining reaction, which is a good negative control. (5) The primary antibody can be replaced by non-immune serum, but this is less specific than the preabsorption method. (6) When an antibody is used for the first time, several dilutions have to be tested against a constant concentration of the secondary antibody in order to establish the lowest working concentration of the primary antibody that gives reproducible and specific results. Finally, the specificity of the secondary antibody is tested by omitting the primary antibody.

TUNEL

Apoptosis is a programmed cell death with special characteristics. The hallmark of apoptosis is DNA fragmentation. At the early stages of apoptosis, extensive non-random fragmentation of DNA occurs. Cleavage of the DNA may yield double-stranded, low-molecular-weight DNA fragments (mono- and oligonucleosomes). The main method to detect apoptotic chondrocytes in growth plates is the TUNEL method. This method is widely used, and it is well described in studies of growth plate apoptosis. Briefly, TUNEL detects blunt ends of double-stranded DNA, an indication of DNA fragmentation by enzymatic (terminal transferase) labeling of the free 3′-OH terminal modified nucleotides. The modified nucleotides can be labeled with peroxidase, digoxigenin, or fluorescent for the development of color. However, the experimental conditions, mainly during the digestion with proteinase-K, can give false positive results and label cells that are not really apoptotic.

As an example, during proliferation where the DNA opens for replication, there are blunt ends of double-stranded DNA (Okazaki phenomenon) as the replication of the DNA proceeds. This could explain why many studies find that numerous proliferative as well as hypertrophic chondrocytes are TUNEL positive. Based on reported studies as well as in a series of pivotal experiments, we optimized the conditions of proteinase-K digestion which is a crucial step during the assay procedure. We found that 10 min of incubation with proteinase-K (20 μg/ml) instead of the manufacturer's recommendation of 20 min gives no false positive results based on the morphology of the nuclear labeling in chondrocytes [14]. In sections from cultured metatarsal bones, the experimental protocol has to be further modified and the concentration of proteinase-K has to be decreased to 5 μg/ml in order to avoid the false positive staining [15].

Organ Culture

Fetal Rat Metatarsal Culture

In vivo experiments on growth plates can give valuable information, but the amount of tissue is limited as well as the methodological options. In addition, growth plates from in vivo experiments are affected not only by local but also systemic factors. Therefore, in vitro models can be helpful in eliminating some of the problems arising when experiments are performed in whole animals and separate the systemic and local effects of different factors. The model of metatarsal organ culture can eliminate the effect of systemic factors and provide information about the effects of different factors and experimental conditions locally in the growth plate. The unique feature of this model is that, like in the in vivo situation, chondrocytes in different phases of chondrogenesis are surrounded by cartilage matrix and are in direct contact with each other, a condition which is absent in cell lines in culture. Thus, compared to using cultured cells, organ culture has the advantage of providing conditions closer to the in vivo situation, making the results easier to extrapolate.

Most of the protocols for the metatarsal organ culture model use the three middle metatarsal bones from the hind legs of rat fetuses (embryonic day 20) [15]. They are dissected, transferred to 24-well plates, one bone per well, in appropriate medium. The length of each metatarsal can be measured by using a digital camera attached to a dissecting microscope at certain time points. The metatarsals from E20 have the structure of a growth plate with the epiphyseal region corresponding to the resting zone, proliferative and HZs and at the middle the primary ossification center (fig. 3).

Postnatal Rat Metatarsal Culture

Postnatal rat metatarsal culture can be used to delineate mechanisms of postnatal growth; fetal and postnatal growth is regulated differently, at least in humans [16]. Compared to studies using fetal bones, the results obtained using a postnatal

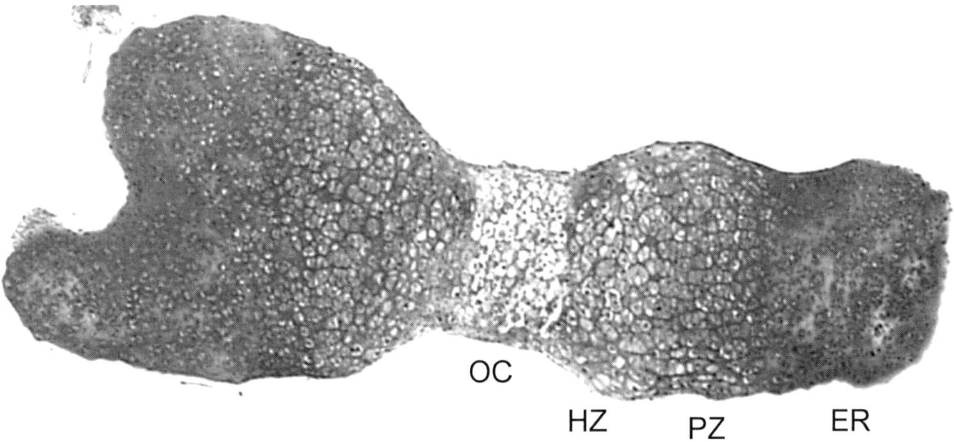

Fig. 3. Cultured fetal rat metatarsal stained with Alcian blue. ER = Epiphyseal region; OC = ossification center.

metatarsal model better reflect the normal physiology and the regulation of postnatal growth in vivo.

Human Fetal Epiphyseal Cartilage and Chondrocyte Biology: Developmental and Clinical Applications

The study of human growth plate biology at the sequential developmental stages and the analysis of the pathophysiology of the widely varying causes of growth retardation are hampered by the difficulty in obtaining fresh material in adequate quantities.

Analysis of whole tissue sections allowed us to show abnormal morphometry in two different fetal entities: the anencephalic fetus and the 21-trisomic fetus [17, 18]. For several years, we have been using the model of human chondrocytes obtained from fetal epiphyseal cartilages to characterize their in vitro regulation by different hormones and growth factors (mainly androgens, estrogens, thyroid hormones, somatostatin, TGF-β, VEGF, IGF-I, GH, glucocorticoids and vitamin D) [19–22]. At our centre, we have obtained fresh material after the corresponding informed consents and suitability for establishing primary cell cultures. This material was available through the Vall d'Hebron Fetal Tissue Bank (Barcelona, Spain) to researchers (within and outside the Institution) as fresh (mostly restricted to in-house studies), frozen and paraffin-embedded sections including both normal and abnormal diagnoses. This constitutes an invaluable resource for the scientific community to develop research in the field of normal growth and abnormal skeletal growth with an impact on fetal life and thereafter.

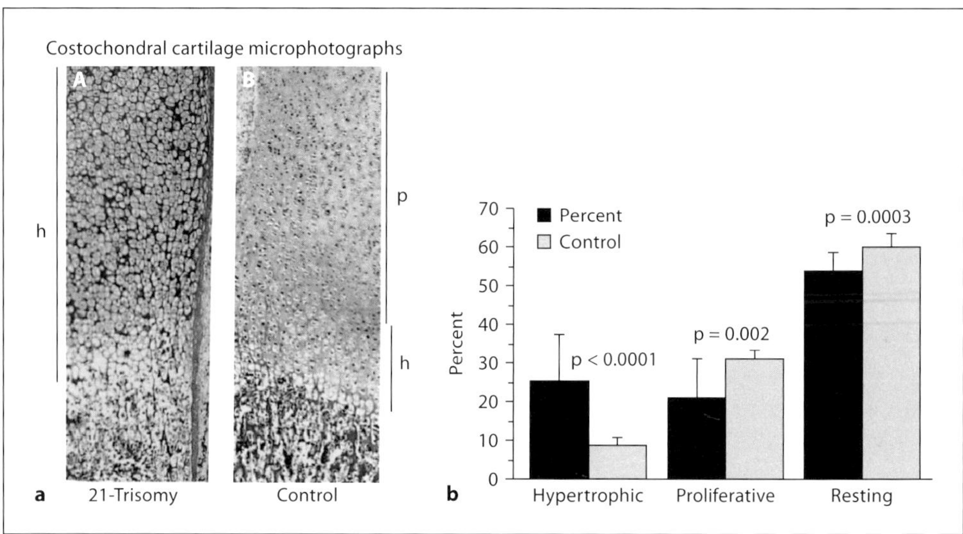

Fig. 4. **a** Comparison of an identical length of trisomy-21 (**A**) and control (**B**) costochondral junctions in the fetal rib including HZ (h) in **A** and **B** and PZ (p) in **B**. HE. ×25. **b** Percentage of total growth cartilage length in each zone (resting, proliferative and hypertrophic; mean ± SD) in ribs from human fetuses with Down's syndrome or other entities not affecting longitudinal skeletal growth (control).

Several human chondrocytic cell lines have been obtained and have proved to be suitable for chondrocyte biology analysis under varied experimental conditions [23].

Human Fetal Rib Morphometry

Human fetal costochondral cartilage histopathological sections can be used for morphometric description and measurement. Ribs (4th and 5th) were obtained from normal (GA = 16–22 weeks; n = 20), anencephalic (GA = 18–22 weeks; n = 8) and 21-trisomic human fetuses (GA = 17–22 weeks; n = 16) and processed as described [17, 18] to measure the lengths and cell densities of resting, proliferative, maturing and HZs. The comparison of anencephalic and 21-trisomic fetuses (fig. 4) with normal fetuses demonstrated that significant differences existed in both [17, 18].

Human Fetal Epiphyseal Cartilage Chondrocyte Culture

Tibial and femoral epiphyseal cartilage from human fetuses, products of legal terminations, was collected with informed parental consent within 12 h post-mortem.

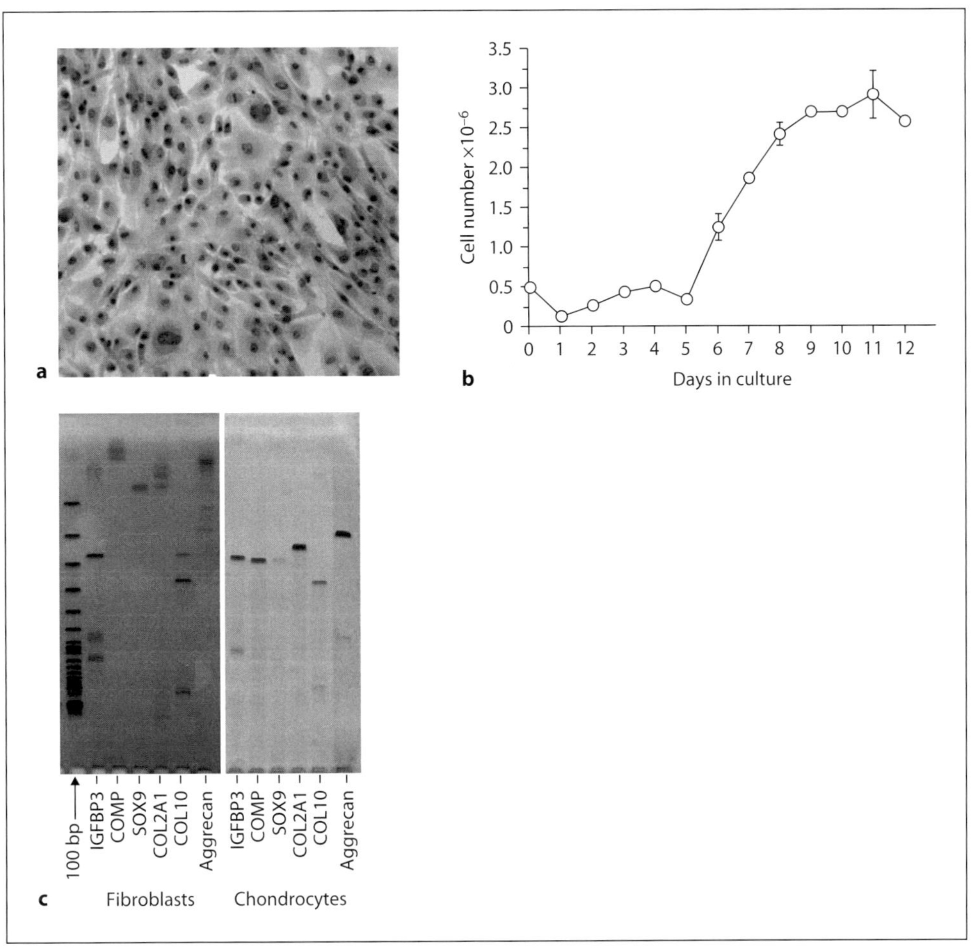

Fig. 5. **a** Human fetal epiphyseal chondrocytes in primary culture. HE. ×10. **b** Cell growth curve (mean ± SD of 3 flasks). **c** Gel electrophoresis of chondrocyte phenotype genes in human fetal epiphyseal chondrocytes as compared with fetal skin fibroblasts: chondrocytes express COMP, SOX9, Col2A1, Aggrecan and even COL10, whereas fibroblasts do not; both express IGFBP-3.

The protocol was approved by the Hospital Ethics Committee. Only fetuses with normal karyotype and diagnoses which do not affect skeletal growth were retained. The epiphyseal cartilage was cleaned of surrounding tissue under sterile conditions. The remaining cartilage was cut into thin slices and finely chopped with a surgical blade. Chondrocytes were released by enzymatic digestion and cultured as previously described [19]. Briefly, a chondrocyte suspension was obtained after enzymatic digestion with trypsin and collagenase. Approximately 4,000–7,000 cells/cm^2 were plated in a 75-cm^2 plastic culture flask with 12 ml of Ham F-12 medium. The culture media were supplemented with 10% FCS and 25 IU/ml of penicillin and streptomycin. The flasks were maintained at 37°C in an atmosphere of 5% CO_2 in humid air. The cultures were fed by changing the medium every 3 days (fig. 5).

Human C-28/I2 Chondrocytic Cell Line Culture

The immortalized human chondrocyte C-28/I2 cell line was established by Goldring et al. [23]. These cells, derived from juvenile costal cartilage, express the differentiated chondrocyte phenotypic markers of type II collagen and aggrecan, but not the hypertrophic chondrocyte marker, type X collagen.

Cultures are maintained in a 5% CO_2 incubator at 37°C in DMEM supplemented with 10% FCS. Chondrocytes are seeded at a density of 75,000 cells/cm^2 in 25 cm^2 plates. Every day, for 14 days, three plates are trypsinized, cell number counted and a pellet of cells from the three plates frozen and stored at –80°C until use. In the culture conditions used, exponential proliferation is observed between days 5 and 10 and confluence is maintained from day 10 to 12 (fig. 6).

Cell Proliferation Analysis following ^{3}H-Thymidine Incorporation into DNA

This method has previously been described [19–22]. Briefly, primary confluent chondrocytes are trypsinized and plated in 96-microwell tissue culture plates at a density of 60,000 cells/cm^2, in 0.3 ml Ham F-12 serum- and antibiotic-free medium. After 48 h, medium is aspirated, and chondrocytes are incubated for 48 h under the different experimental conditions. [^{3}H]-thymidine (5 μCi/ml) is added for the last 24 h of incubation. Four different wells are prepared for each condition. Results for each condition are expressed as percent of mean radioactivity in four wells with respect to the control condition (100%). Proliferation rate is measured as the index of ^{3}H-thymidine incorporation into DNA with the different experimental conditions.

Gene Expression Analysis in Human Fetal Epiphyseal Chondrocytes

For gene expression study, primary confluent chondrocytes are trypsinized and 42,000 cells/cm^2 plated in 6-well tissue culture plates with 2 ml Ham F-12 serum- and antibiotic-free medium. After 48 h, this medium is aspirated and chondrocytes incubated for 48 h under different experimental conditions. Cells are trypsinized and 350 μl of guanidine isothiocyanate solution added to the pellet.

Total RNA is isolated, and cDNA synthesis analyzed as previously described [21, 22]. For Taqman-based real-time PCR expression profiling, 0.4 μl of each cDNA (2 μl for IGF-I gene quantitation) is added to the Taqman Universal PCR Master Mix along with Assays-on-Demand® according to the manufacturer's (Applied Biosystems) instructions in a total volume of 20 μl. Assays-on-Demand are used to quantify gene expression (http://products.appliedbiosystems.com). The huCYC is selected as a reference gene using TaqMan Human Endogenous Control Plate (Applied Biosystems).

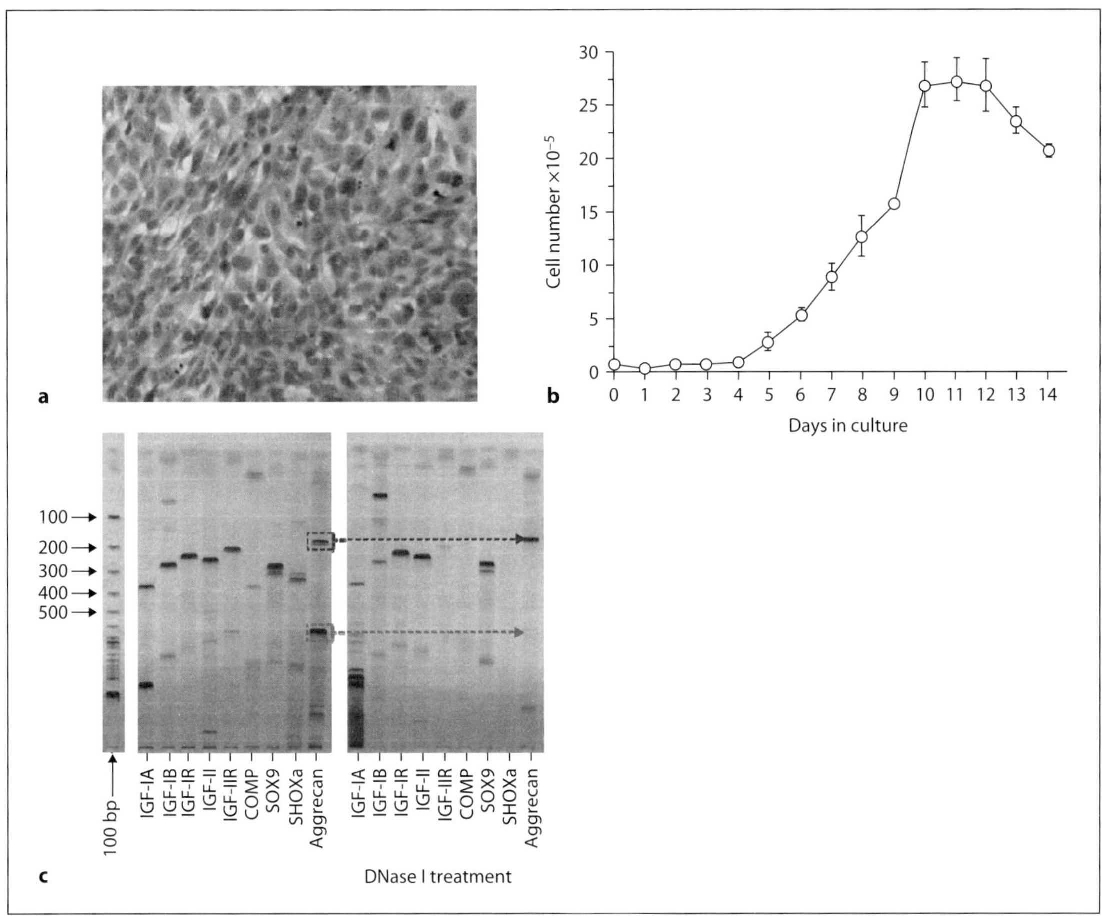

Fig. 6. a Human chondrocytic cell line C-28/I2 culture. HE. ×10. **b** Cell growth curve (mean ± SD of 3 flasks). Under culture conditions used, exponential proliferation was observed between days 5 and 10, and confluency was maintained from day 10 to 12. **c** Gel electrophoresis of IGF axis genes (IGF-IA and IGF-IB, IGF-II, IGF1R and IGFIIR) and chondrocytic phenotype markers (SOX9, SHOXa, COMP and aggrecan).

Real-time fluorescence is monitored using the ABI PRISM 7000 instrument. Relative expression levels of the various transcripts are generated and the relative abundance then determined by comparing the C_t values for each reaction with the comparative C_t method ($2^{\Delta\Delta Ct}$) with the control condition. Variations in input cDNA mass are corrected by normalizing all data with the corresponding huCYC levels. All measurements are performed in triplicate.

References

1 Sandberg M, Vuorio E: Localization of types I, II, and III collagen mRNAs in developing human skeletal tissues by in situ hybridization. J Cell Biol 1987;104:1077–1084.

2 Horton WA: Skeletal development: insights from targeting the mouse genome. Lancet 2003;362:560–569.

3 Kuettner KE, Pauli BU, Gall G, Memoli VA, Schenk RK: Synthesis of cartilage matrix by mammalian chondrocytes in vitro. I. Isolation, culture characteristics, and morphology. J Cell Biol 1982;93:743–750.

4 Ballock RT, Reddi AH: Thyroxine is the serum factor that regulates morphogenesis of columnar cartilage from isolated chondrocytes in chemically defined medium. J Cell Biol 1994;126:1311–1318.

5 Hoemann CD, El-Gabalawy H, McKee MD: In vitro osteogenesis assays: influence of the primary cell source on alkaline phosphatase activity and mineralization. Pathol Biol (Paris) 2009;57:318–323.

6 Nilsson O, Parker EA, Hegde A, Chau M, Barnes KM, Baron J: Gradients in bone morphogenetic protein-related gene expression across the growth plate. J Endocrinol 2007;193:75–84.

7 Andrade AC, Nilsson O, Barnes KM, Baron J: Wnt gene expression in the post-natal growth plate: regulation with chondrocyte differentiation. Bone 2007;40:1361–1369.

8 Lui JC, Andrade AC, Forcinito P, Hegde A, Chen W, Baron J, Nilsson O: Spatial and temporal regulation of gene expression in the mammalian growth plate. Bone 2010;46:1380–1390.

9 van Buul S, Van den Brande J: The Snell-dwarfmouse. I. General growth pattern, before and during growth hormone and thyroxine therapy. Acta Endocrinol (Copenh) 1978;89:632–645.

10 Heinrichs C, Yanovski JA, Roth AH, Yu YM, Domene HM, Yano K, Cutler GB Jr., Baron J: Dexamethasone increases growth hormone receptor messenger ribonucleic acid levels in liver and growth plate. Endocrinology 1994;135:1113–1118.

11 Andrade AC, Lui JC, Nilsson O: Temporal and spatial expression of a growth-regulated network of imprinted genes in growth plate. Pediatr Nephrol 2010;25:617–623.

12 Chrysis D, Ritzen EM, Savendahl L: Growth retardation induced by dexamethasone is associated with increased apoptosis of the growth plate chondrocytes. J Endocrinol 2003;176:331–337.

13 Taylor CR: Paraffin section immunocytochemistry for estrogen receptor: the time has come. Cancer 1996;77:2419–2422.

14 Chrysis D, Nilsson O, Ritzen EM, Savendahl L: Apoptosis is developmentally regulated in rat growth plate. Endocrine 2002;18:271–278.

15 Martensson K, Chrysis D, Savendahl L: Interleukin-1beta and TNF-alpha act in synergy to inhibit longitudinal growth in fetal rat metatarsal bones. J Bone Miner Res 2004;19:1805–1812.

16 Chagin AS, Karimian E, Sundstrom K, Eriksson E, Savendahl L: Catch-up growth after dexamethasone withdrawal occurs in cultured postnatal rat metatarsal bones. J Endocrinol 2010;204:21–29.

17 Garcia-Ramirez M, Toran N, Carrascosa A, Audi L: Anomalous costochondral cartilage in fetal anencephaly. Pediatr Dev Pathol 2000;3:256–263.

18 Garcia-Ramirez M, Toran N, Carrascosa A, Audi L: Down's syndrome: altered chondrogenesis in fetal rib. Pediatr Res 1998;44:93–98.

19 Carrascosa A, Audi L, Ballabriga A: Morphologic and metabolic development of human fetal epiphyseal chondrocytes in primary culture. Pediatr Res 1985;19:720–727.

20 Garcia-Ramirez M, Audi L, Andaluz P, Carrascosa A: Effects of TGF-beta1 on proliferation and IGFbp-3 production in a primary culture of human fetal epiphyseal chondrocytes (HFEC). J Clin Endocrinol Metab 1999;84:2978–2981.

21 Fernandez-Cancio M, Esteban C, Carrascosa A, Toran N, Andaluz P, Audi L: IGF-I and not IGF-II expression is regulated by glucocorticoids in human fetal epiphyseal chondrocytes. Growth Horm IGF Res 2008;18:497–505.

22 Fernandez-Cancio M, Audi L, Carrascosa A, Toran N, Andaluz P, Esteban C, Granada ML: Vitamin d and growth hormone regulate growth hormone/insulin-like growth factor (GH-IGF) axis gene expression in human fetal epiphyseal chondrocytes. Growth Horm IGF Res 2009;19:232–237.

23 Goldring MB, Birkhead JR, Suen LF, Yamin R, Mizuno S, Glowacki J, Arbiser JL, Apperley JF: Interleukin-1 beta-modulated gene expression in immortalized human chondrocytes. J Clin Invest 1994;94:2307–2316.

Dr. Anenisia C. Andrade
Pediatric Endocrinology Unit, Q2:08, Department of Women's and Children's Health
Karolinska Institutet and Karolinska University Hospital
SE–171 76 Stockholm (Sweden)
Tel. +46 8 5177 6530, E-Mail anenisia@gmail.com

Camacho-Hübner C, Nilsson O, Sävendahl L (eds): Cartilage and Bone Development and Its Disorders.
Endocr Dev. Basel, Karger, 2011, vol 21, pp 67–77

Fibroblast Growth Factor-23 and Phosphorus Metabolism

Dov Tiosano

Pediatric Endocrinology, Meyer Children's Hospital, Rambam Medical Center, Rappaport Family Faculty of Medicine, Technion-Israel Institute of Technology, Haifa, Israel

Abstract

The understanding of phosphorus metabolism has expanded considerably over the last decade. Recent studies have identified a novel bone-kidney endocrine axis that maintains phosphate homeostasis. When phosphate is in excess, FGF-23 is secreted from bone and acts on the kidney to promote phosphate excretion into urine and to suppress vitamin D synthesis, thereby inducing negative phosphate balance. This review summarizes the role of the FGF-23 axis on phosphorus metabolism, and presents the clinical entities that arise from activation or inactivation of the FGF-23 axis.

Plasma phosphorous (Pi) levels are maintained in a very narrow range. They are higher during infancy (4.5–8.3 mg/dl or 1.5–2.65 mM) and childhood (3.7–5.6 mg/dl or 1.5–2.65 mM) than during puberty and adulthood (2.5–4.5 mg/dl or 0.9–1.5 mM) [1].

The skeleton and muscles, the principal Pi reservoir in the body, comprise approximately 80% of the total body Pi, the remainder being in soft tissues and extracellular fluids. Of Pi filtered in the kidneys, 80–90% is re-adsorbed in the proximal tubule. In adults, the average amount of Pi excreted is almost equivalent to that absorbed in the intestines. During periods of rapid growth and development in infancy and in puberty, a positive phosphate balance is established. The complex homeostasis of Pi absorption is controlled by Pi itself, and by calcitriol, PTH, and FGF-23, through coordinated function of several organ systems [2]. Calcitriol regulates Pi absorption in the intestines mainly by the type II cotransporter NaPi-IIb, which is not expressed in the kidney [3]. In the osteoblast, calcitriol and phosphorus have positive effects on the generation and secretion of FGF-23, while PTH is responsible for the release of Pi from the bone [4].

Renal handling of Pi is regulated by hormonal and nonhormonal factors. The three main factors that regulate Pi re-adsorption by the sodium/Pi cotransporter in the proximal tubule are: urinary Pi, PTH, and FGF-23. Changes in urinary excretion of Pi are almost invariably mirrored by changes in the apical expression of NaPi-IIa and NaPi-IIc in proximal tubules. Phosphate deprivation increases NaPi-IIa and NaPi-IIc expression, which enhances phosphorus absorption. PTH, FGF-23, and dietary phosphate regulate NaPi-IIa and NaPi-IIc similarly. PTH and FGF-23 accelerate the cotransporter endocytosis, while FGF-23 also accelerates cotransporter degradation in the lysosome and reduces NaPi-IIa and NaPi-IIc expression [5].

Fibroblast Growth Factor-23

FGF-23 is a 30-kDa protein that is proteolytically processed to generate smaller NH_2-terminal (18 kDa) and COOH-terminal (12 kDa) fragments. The NH_2-terminal fragment of FGF-23 contains the FGFR-binding domain.

FGF-23 functions principally as a phosphaturic factor [6]. It is secreted by osteocytes and osteoblasts in response to high serum phosphate levels and to 1,25(OH)2D_3 [3, 7]. The net secretion of an intact FGF-23 protein and split FGF-23 depends on the balance between the activity of GALNT 3 that prevents its degradation, and the subtilisin/furine-like endopeptidases that degrade FGF-23. In the osteoblast, FGF-23 posttranslation undergoes O-glycosylation by GALNT 3; the glycosylation protects the molecule from degradation. Nonglycosylated FGF-23 may be targeted for degradation by subtilisin/furine-like endopeptidases (fig. 1). Impaired FGF-23 synthesis or action, due to FGF-23 gene mutations, mutations in GALNT 3, or mutations in Klotho, which is required for the conversion of FGFR1(IIIc) into the FGF-23 receptor, lead to severe hyperphosphatemia and tumoral calcinosis (fig. 2) [8–10].

FGF-23 inhibits renal phosphate reabsorption by NaPi-2a and NaPi-2c cotransporters, thereby increasing urinary phosphate excretion [11]. In addition, FGF-23 suppresses 1α-hydroxylase expression, resulting in reduced production of the active vitamin D metabolite 1,25(OH)2D_3. Thus, the hallmark of all clinical entities that share high FGF-23 activity is rickets/osteomalacia, hypophosphatemia due to renal phosphate wasting and low 1,25(OH)2D_3 levels. Moreover, FGF-23 can also induce 24-hydroxylase, which degrades 1,25(OH)2D_3 (55). Since 1,25(OH)2D_3 can enhance intestinal phosphate absorption, FGF-23 expression attenuates intestinal phosphate absorption by reducing 1α-hydroxylase. The FGF-23-mediated regulation of phosphate homeostasis is in large part independent of calcium homeostasis; for its action, FGF-23 needs the coreceptor Klotho.

In Greek mythology, life span is controlled by the three daughters of Zeus and Themis, namely Klotho, who combs and spins the thread of life, Lachesis, who determines the length of life by measuring the length of thread, and Athropos who cuts the string to bring life to an end.

Klotho was conferred to a gene that was fortuitously discovered in 1997. Klotho mutant mice were originally described as a short-lived model that displays a variety

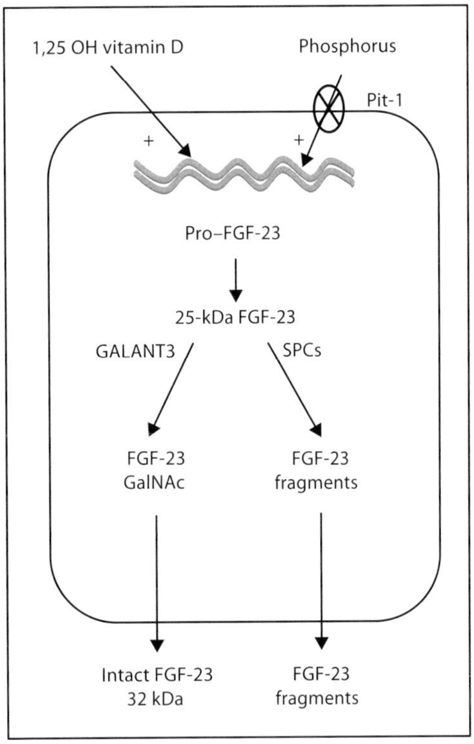

1,25 OH vitamin D

Phosphorus

Pit-1

+ +

Pro–FGF-23

25-kDa FGF-23

GALANT3 SPCs

FGF-23 GalNAc

FGF-23 fragments

Intact FGF-23 32 kDa

FGF-23 fragments

Fig. 1. Hyperphosphatemia and 1,25 OH vitamin D lead to the secretion of FGF-23. Phosphorus enters the cell through the Pit-1 transporter. The net secretion of an intact FGF-23 depends on the balanced activity of GALNT 3, which prevents FGF-23 degradation, and on the subtilisin/furine-like endopeptidases (SPCs) that degrade FGF-23. In the osteoblast, FGF-23 undergoes posttranslation modification, O-glycosylation, by GALNT 3; the glycosylation protects the molecule from degradation. Nonglycosylated FGF-23 may be targeted for degradation by subtilisin/furine-like endopeptidases.

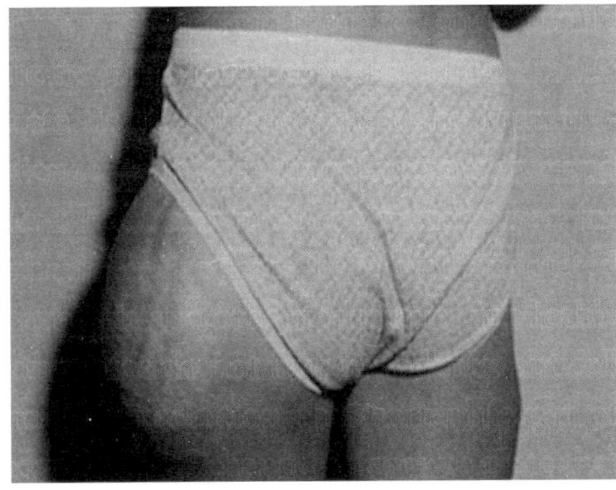

Fig. 2. Tumoral calcinosis. Mutations in GALANT3, FGF-23, and Klotho were found in patients with tumoral calcinosis.

of premature aging-related phenotypes, such as arteriosclerosis, ectopic calcification in various soft tissues, decreased bone mineral density, uncoordinated movement, atrophy of the skin, and severe hyperphosphatemia associated with increased concentrations of 1,25(OH)2D_3 [12].

The *klotho* gene encodes a type 1 membrane protein, which is predicted to be present on the cell surface of Klotho-expressing cells. The human *klotho* gene has five exons and can generate two transcripts. The full-length transcript is 5.2 kb and encodes a 130-kDa membrane protein. Once its short transmembrane domain is removed, this membrane form can be released into circulation. A disintegrin and metalloproteinases (ADAM-10 and ADAM-17) are capable of cleavage of Klotho from the plasma membrane [13].

Klotho expression has been detected mostly in the distal convoluted tubules of the kidney, the parathyroid gland, and the epithelium of the choroid plexus in the brain [14]. In the kidney, α-Klotho is exclusively coexpressed with calcium-permeable TRPV5 channels. Chang et al. [15] reported a novel mechanism that regulates the abundance of TRPV5 at the luminal cell surface: α-Klotho in urine, as a β-glucuronidase, increases TRPV5 channel abundance at the luminal cell surface by hydrolyzing the N-linked extracellular sugar residues of TRPV5.

Parathyroid glands play a key role in systemic calcium homeostasis. These glands express both FGFR1 and Klotho. FGF-23 decreases parathyroid hormone gene expression and hormone secretion directly, causing the parathyroid to activate the MAPK pathway and to decrease PTH secretion. The finding that FGF-23 decreases PTH gene expression and secretion contrasts with the parallel increase in both FGF-23 and serum PTH observed in renal failure. Canalejo et al. [16] have shown that the parathyroid cells in uremic patients resist the inhibitory effects of FGF-23, partly due to depressed expression of FGFR1 and Klotho in this condition.

Sodium Phosphorus Symporters in the Osteocyte

The process of osteoblast differentiation and matrix mineralization requires alkaline phosphatase (ALP) enzymatic activity, which generates free Pi. ALP is localized to the plasma membrane and oriented such that its catalytic subunit is ectoplasmic. Within the extracellular environment, ALP cleaves a phosphate from β-glycerol phosphate to release free glycerol and form pyrophosphate. The free Pi enters the cell through an Na-dependent phosphate transporter and regulates gene transcription and cellular function [17, 18]. Intracellular Pi is maintained within a narrow range, and is a rate-limiting step in osteocyte mineralization.

Low levels of Pi transported via Pit-1 stimulate stanniocalcin 1 (STC1) and ALP expression. STC1, acting as an autocrine/paracrine factor, induces Pit-1 expression directly, increasing Pi transport. At the same time, ALP, by its action on β-glycerol phosphate, maintains normal intracellular phosphate in the osteoblast, and normal osteopontin expression [19]. The latter facilitates the attachment of osteoblasts and osteoclasts to the extracellular matrix and modulates hydroxyapatite crystal elongation during bone formation. In the hypophosphatemic state, this mechanism does not compensate for the low phosphorus levels in the osteoblast, thus explaining why ALP levels remain elevated until serum phosphate levels are corrected (fig. 3).

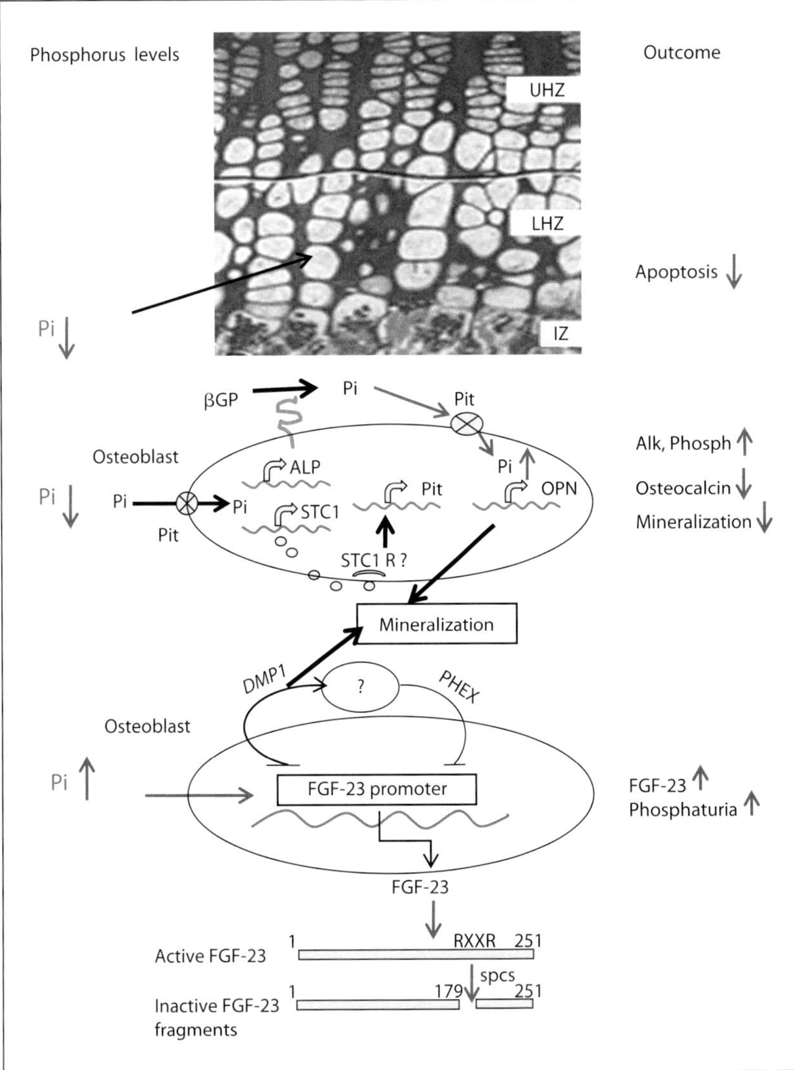

Fig. 3. Effects of hypophosphatemia and hyperphosphatemia on bone. In the growth plate, hypophosphatemia causes arrest of apoptosis in hypertrophic chondrocytes, leading to rickets. In osteoblasts, hypophosphatemia inhibits maturation and mineralization leading to osteomalacia. In the presence of high phosphorus, FGF-23 is secreted, promoting phosphaturia and normalizing phosphorus.

FGF-23 as the Osteoblast Pi Threshold Keeper

While ALP and STC1 secretion protect cells from low Pi levels, FGF-23 appears to protect cells from hyperphosphatemia. Hyperphosphatemia negatively impacts osteoblasts; overloading of Pi causes cell death. NaPi transport stimulation above a critical threshold, as occurs with extracellular Pi above 5 mM, is evident in FGF-23-null mice [20–22].

Studies in Hyp mice (the murine analogue of X-linked hypophosphatemia) provide indirect evidence of the relationship between high Pi levels and FGF23 secretion. In Hyp mice, FGF-23 is 5- to 25-fold higher than in normal mice. However, when dietary Pi is reduced, FGF-23 concentration decreases by more than 3-fold, with levels correlating directly with those of serum Pi [4]. In concordance with these findings, when hyperphosphatemia presents due to reduced PTH secretion following partial thyroidectomy, serum levels of FGF-23 are elevated. FGF-23 levels normalize after recovery of parathyroid function and normalization of serum Pi levels. The peak level of serum phosphorus always precedes that of FGF-23 by several days, suggesting that elevated Pi is a primary stimulus for release of FGF-23 [23]. The significant effect of dietary phosphorus on serum FGF-23 concentrations was demonstrated by the considerably higher levels of FGF-23 measured following high-normal Pi dietary intake (2,300 mg/day) compared with those following low-normal Pi dietary intake (625 mg/day) [24]. In patients with elevated serum phosphorus due to renal function decline, the circulating concentration of FGF-23 increases [25]. This indirect evidence ascribes FGF-23 the role of maintaining a phosphorus threshold that protects osteoblasts from high phosphorus levels.

Rickets due to High FGF-23

Causes for high FGF-23 include overproduction by osteocytes, bone tumor or bone fibrous dysplasia, degradation defect of FGF-23 through increased Klotho production, and end organ gain of function.

Increased FGF-23 Production by Osteocytes

X-linked hypophosphatemic rickets (XLHR) is a dominant disorder characterized by impaired phosphate uptake in the kidney. XLHR is caused by inactivating mutations in PHEX that lead to increased circulating FGF-23 levels [26].

Autosomal recessive hypophosphatemia rickets (ARHR) is caused by inactivating mutations in DMP1, a member of the small integrin-binding ligand N-linked glycoprotein family of extracellular matrix proteins that augment mineralization. Loss of function of DMP1 results in increased transcription of FGF-23 by osteocytes [27].

Recently, Lorenz-Depiereux et al. [29] found that mutations in ectonucleotide pyrophosphatase/phosphodiesterase 1 (ENPP1), beside generalized arterial calcification (GACI) of infancy [28], are associated with abnormally elevated FGF-23, that leads to hypophosphatemic rickets without GACI. An explanation is lacking for the phenotypic differences between patients with *enpp1* mutations; in some, hypophosphatemic rickets appears, while in others generalized arterial calcification develops. Interestingly, the same homozygous *enpp1* mutation can result in different phenotypes.

Decreased FGF-23 Degradation

Autosomal dominant hypophosphatemic rickets, caused by mutations (R176Q and R179W) in the RXXR furin-like cleavage domain of FGF-23, impairs proteolytic inactivation of FGF-23 [30].

Increased FGF-23 Production by Tumors and Fibrous Lesions

Polyostotic fibrous dysplasia (PFD), also called McCune-Albright syndrome, is caused by an activating mutation in the guanine nucleotide binding protein, α-stimulating gene *(GNAS1)*, and results in fibrodysplastic tissue. In some patients, hypophosphatemia results from elevated levels of circulating FGF-23 [31].

Tumor-induced osteomalacia, or oncogenic osteomalacia, is a paraneoplastic syndrome of renal phosphate wasting, aberrant vitamin D metabolism, and osteomalacia that is associated with elevated FGF-23 levels [32]. Both PFD and tumor-induced osteomalacia disorders are associated with increased levels of MEPE and sFRP4, which regulate PHEX and DMP1 metabolism [33].

Increased FGF-23 due to Increased Klotho Production

The association of hyperparathyroidism and rickets has been reported, but remains controversial. Some patients had parathyroid gland adenoma, while others had hyperplasia [34]. Brownstein et al. [35] investigated a patient with hypophosphatemic rickets and hyperparathyroidism and found that it was due to a de novo translocation with a breakpoint adjacent to α-Klotho, which encodes a β-glucuronidase. Plasma α-Klotho levels, β-glucuronidase activity, and circulating FGF-23 levels were markedly elevated.

FGFR1, FGFR2, and FGFR3 Mutations

In vitro studies indicate that the N-terminal region of FGF-23 binds to and activates FGFR1, -3, and -4. In cases where mutations occur in these receptors, FGF-23 is elevated and may lead to rickets.

Linear Sebaceous or Epidermal Nevus Syndrome
There have been a number of reports of the association of hypophosphatemic rickets with epidermal nevus caused by a mosaicism of activating FGFR3 mutations in the human epidermis. Some of these patients presented with ipsilateral focal bone disease associated with hypophosphatemic rickets, elevated circulating FGF-23 levels, and aberrant 1,25(OH)2D_3 levels, similar to other syndromes caused by elevated FGF-23 [36].

Osteoglophonic Dysplasia
Osteoglophonic dysplasia is a rare disorder with a skeletal phenotype associated with FGFR1, FGFR2, and FGFR3 mutations that may regulate FGF-23 expression in bone or in the renal handling of phosphate [37]. Patients with osteoglophonic dysplasia present with craniosynostosis, prominent supraorbital ridge, and a depressed nasal bridge.

FGF-23 and Tumoral Calcinosis

Tumoral calcinosis is characterized by the presence of ectopic calcifications around major joints

The GALNT3 gene encodes GalNAc-T3, which prevents degradation of FGF-23, thereby allowing secretion of intact FGF-23. Biallelic mutations in either GALNT3 or FGF-23 result in hyperphosphatemic familial tumoral calcinosis or its variant, hyperostosis-hyperphosphatemia syndrome.

Under normal physiological circumstances, hyperphosphatemia and FGF-23 inhibit renal 1,25(OH)2D_3 synthesis, thereby leading to low 1,25(OH)2D_3 levels. However, compromised FGF-23 signaling, due to mutations in any of the 3 genes involved in tumoral calcinosis (FGF-23, GALNT3, and KL), disrupts this negative feedback mechanism, resulting in increased serum 1,25(OH)2D_3 concentrations and hyperphosphatemia.

Tumoral calcinosis patients with inactivating mutations in FGF-23 or GALNT3 have highly elevated C-terminal fragments but low or undetectable levels of intact (active) FGF-23 [38, 39]. In these cases, FGF-23 production is increased to compensate for hyperphosphatemia, but the FGF-23 protein is unstable and readily cleaved by intracellular furin-like convertases. Whereas mutation in the *klotho* gene elevates intact and C-terminal FGF-23 levels as expected, the reduced capability of mutant klotho to form a ternary FGF-23-kl-fgfr1c complex comprises FGF-23 signaling.

The common metabolic features in tumoral calcinosis are hyperphosphatemia, abnormally elevated 1,25(OH)2D_3, and PTH.

Conclusions

The common denominator of all rickets is hypophosphatemia. Hypophosphatemia prevents apoptosis in the hypertrophic cells in the growth plate. The result is accumulation of hypertrophic cells in the growth plate, forming the rachitic bone. Diagnosis of rickets should thus be based on the etiologies of hypophosphatemia.

The three major entities that can lead to hypophosphatemia are high PTH activity, high FGF-23 activity, and renal defects that lead to Pi wasting. Hallmarks of high PTH activity are: hypophosphatemia, phosphaturia, disturbance in vitamin D metabolism, and low calcium. Hallmarks of high FGF-23 activity are hypophosphatemia and phosphaturia, with inappropriately low 1,25 OH2D. Hallmarks of renal rickets are hypophosphatemia and phosphaturia with high 1,25 OH2D resulting in hypercalciuria.

References

1 Hochberg Z: Abnormalities of Calcium and Parathyroid Hormone. Philadelphia, Lippincott Williams and Wilkins, 2004.

2 Quarles LD: Endocrine functions of bone in mineral metabolism regulation. J Clin Invest 2008;118: 3820–3828.

3 Rizzoli R, Fleisch H, Bonjour JP: Role of 1,25-dihydroxyvitamin D3 on intestinal phosphate absorption in rats with a normal vitamin D supply. J Clin Invest 1977;60:639–647.

4 Perwad F, Azam N, Zhang MY, Yamashita T, Tenenhouse HS, Portale AA: Dietary and serum phosphorus regulate fibroblast growth factor 23 expression and 1,25-dihydroxyvitamin D metabolism in mice. Endocrinology 2005;146:5358–5364.

5 Murer H, Hernando N, Forster I, Biber J: Proximal tubular phosphate reabsorption: molecular mechanisms. Physiol Rev 2000;80:1373–1409.

6 Shimada T, Mizutani S, Muto T, Yoneya T, Hino R, Takeda S, Takeuchi Y, Fujita T, Fukumoto S, Yamashita T: Cloning and characterization of FGF-23 as a causative factor of tumor-induced osteomalacia. Proc Natl Acad Sci U S A 2001;98:6500–6505.

7 Kolek OI, Hines ER, Jones MD, LeSueur LK, Lipko MA, Kiela PR, Collins JF, Haussler MR, Ghishan FK: 1alpha,25-Dihydroxyvitamin D3 upregulates FGF-23 gene expression in bone: the final link in a renal-gastrointestinal-skeletal axis that controls phosphate transport. Am J Physiol Gastrointest Liver Physiol 2005;289:G1036–G1042.

8 Garringer HJ, Malekpour M, Esteghamat F, Mortazavi SM, Davis SI, Farrow EG, Yu X, Arking DE, Dietz HC, White KE: Molecular genetic and biochemical analyses of FGF-23 mutations in familial tumoral calcinosis. Am J Physiol Endocrinol Metab 2008;295:E929–E937.

9 Topaz O, Shurman DL, Bergman R, Indelman M, Ratajczak P, Mizrachi M, Khamaysi Z, Behar D, Petronius D, Friedman V, Zelikovic I, Raimer S, Metzker A, Richard G, Sprecher E: Mutations in GALNT3, encoding a protein involved in O-linked glycosylation, cause familial tumoral calcinosis. Nat Genet 2004;36:579–581.

10 Ichikawa S, Imel EA, Kreiter ML, Yu X, Mackenzie DS, Sorenson AH, Goetz R, Mohammadi M, White KE, Econs MJ: A homozygous missense mutation in human KLOTHO causes severe tumoral calcinosis. J Clin Invest 2007;117:2684–2691.

11 Shimada T, Hasegawa H, Yamazaki Y, Muto T, Hino R, Takeuchi Y, Fujita T, Nakahara K, Fukumoto S, Yamashita T: FGF-23 is a potent regulator of vitamin D metabolism and phosphate homeostasis. J Bone Miner Res 2004;19:429–435.

12 Kuro-o M, Matsumura Y, Aizawa H, Kawaguchi H, Suga T, Utsugi T, Ohyama Y, Kurabayashi M, Kaname T, Kume E, Iwasaki H, Iida A, Shiraki-Iida T, Nishikawa S, Nagai R, Nabeshima YI: Mutation of the mouse Klotho gene leads to a syndrome resembling ageing. Nature 1997;390:45–51.

13 Chen CD, Podvin S, Gillespie E, Leeman SE, Abraham CR: Insulin stimulates the cleavage and release of the extracellular domain of Klotho by ADAM10 and ADAM17. Proc Natl Acad Sci U S A 2007;104:19796–19801.

14 Matsumura Y, Aizawa H, Shiraki-Iida T, Nagai R, Kuro-o M, Nabeshima Y: Identification of the human Klotho gene and its two transcripts encoding membrane and secreted Klotho protein. Biochem Biophys Res Commun 1998;242:626–630.
15 Chang Q, Hoefs S, van der Kemp AW, Topala CN, Bindels RJ, Hoenderop JG: The beta-glucuronidase Klotho hydrolyzes and activates the TRPV5 channel. Science 2005;310:490–493.
16 Canalejo R, Canalejo A, Martinez-Moreno JM, Rodriguez-Ortiz ME, Estepa JC, Mendoza FJ, Munoz-Castaneda JR, Shalhoub V, Almaden Y, Rodriguez M FGF-23 fails to inhibit uremic parathyroid glands. J Am Soc Nephrol 2010;21:1125–1135.
17 Beck GR Jr: Inorganic phosphate as a signaling molecule in osteoblast differentiation. J Cell Biochem 2003;90:234–243.
18 Beck GR Jr, Moran E, Knecht N: Inorganic phosphate regulates multiple genes during osteoblast differentiation, including Nrf2. Exp Cell Res 2003; 288:288–300.
19 Beck GR Jr, Zerler B, Moran E: Phosphate is a specific signal for induction of osteopontin gene expression. Proc Natl Acad Sci U S A 2000;97: 8352–8357.
20 Meleti Z, Shapiro IM, Adams CS: Inorganic phosphate induces apoptosis of osteoblast-like cells in culture. Bone 2000;27:359–366.
21 Shimada T, Kakitani M, Yamazaki Y, Hasegawa H, Takeuchi Y, Fujita T, Fukumoto S, Tomizuka K, Yamashita T: Targeted ablation of FGF-23 demonstrates an essential physiological role of FGF-23 in phosphate and vitamin D metabolism. J Clin Invest 2004;113:561–568.
22 Sitara D, Razzaque MS, Hesse M, Yoganathan S, Taguchi T, Erben RG, Juppner H, Lanske B: Homozygous ablation of fibroblast growth factor-23 results in hyperphosphatemia and impaired skeletogenesis, and reverses hypophosphatemia in Phex-deficient mice. Matrix Biol 2004;23:421–432.
23 Yamashita H, Yamazaki Y, Hasegawa H, Yamashita T, Fukumoto S, Shigematsu T, Kazama JJ, Fukagawa M, Noguchi S: Fibroblast growth factor-23 (FGF-23) in patients with transient hypoparathyroidism: its important role in serum phosphate regulation. Endocr J 2007;54:465–470.
24 Antoniucci DM, Yamashita T, Portale AA: Dietary phosphorus regulates serum fibroblast growth factor-23 concentrations in healthy men. J Clin Endocrinol Metab 2006;91:3144–3149.
25 Larsson T, Nisbeth U, Ljunggren O, Juppner H, Jonsson KB: Circulating concentration of FGF-23 increases as renal function declines in patients with chronic kidney disease, but does not change in response to variation in phosphate intake in healthy volunteers. Kidney Int 2003;64:2272–2279.
26 Liu S, Guo R, Simpson LG, Xiao ZS, Burnham CE, Quarles LD: Regulation of fibroblastic growth factor 23 expression but not degradation by PHEX. J Biol Chem 2003;278:37419–37426.
27 Lorenz-Depiereux B, Bastepe M, Benet-Pages A, Amyere M, Wagenstaller J, Muller-Barth U, Badenhoop K, Kaiser SM, Rittmaster RS, Shlossberg AH, Olivares JL, Loris C, Ramos FJ, Glorieux F, Vikkula M, Juppner H, Strom TM: DMP1 mutations in autosomal recessive hypophosphatemia implicate a bone matrix protein in the regulation of phosphate homeostasis. Nat Genet 2006;38:1248–1250.
28 Rutsch F, Ruf N, Vaingankar S, Toliat MR, Suk A, Hohne W, Schauer G, Lehmann M, Roscioli T, Schnabel D, Epplen JT, Knisely A, Superti-Furga A, McGill J, Filippone M, Sinaiko AR, Vallance H, Hinrichs B, Smith W, Ferre M, Terkeltaub R, Nurnberg P: Mutations in ENPP1 are associated with 'idiopathic' infantile arterial calcification. Nat Genet 2003;34:379–381.
29 Lorenz-Depiereux B, Schnabel D, Tiosano D, Hausler G, Strom TM: Loss-of-function ENPP1 mutations cause both generalized arterial calcification of infancy and autosomal-recessive hypophosphatemic rickets. Am J Hum Genet 2010;86: 267–272.
30 Bai XY, Miao D, Goltzman D, Karaplis AC: The autosomal dominant hypophosphatemic rickets R176Q mutation in fibroblast growth factor 23 resists proteolytic cleavage and enhances in vivo biological potency. J Biol Chem 2003;278:9843–9849.
31 Riminucci M, Collins MT, Fedarko NS, Cherman N, Corsi A, White KE, Waguespack S, Gupta A, Hannon T, Econs MJ, Bianco P, Gehron Robey P: FGF-23 in fibrous dysplasia of bone and its relationship to renal phosphate wasting. J Clin Invest 2003; 112:683–692.
32 Jonsson KB, Zahradnik R, Larsson T, White KE, Sugimoto T, Imanishi Y, Yamamoto T, Hampson G, Koshiyama H, Ljunggren O, Oba K, Yang IM, Miyauchi A, Econs MJ, Lavigne J, Juppner H: Fibroblast growth factor 23 in oncogenic osteomalacia and X-linked hypophosphatemia. N Engl J Med 2003;348:1656–1663.

33 Berndt T, Craig TA, Bowe AE, Vassiliadis J, Reczek D, Finnegan R, Jan De Beur SM, Schiavi SC, Kumar R: Secreted frizzled-related protein 4 is a potent tumor-derived phosphaturic agent. J Clin Invest 2003;112:785–794.

34 Menon PS, Madhavi N, Mukhopadhyaya S, Padhy AK, Bal CS, Sharma LK: Primary hyperparathyroidism in a 14 year old girl presenting with bone deformities. J Paediatr Child Health 1994;30:441–443.

35 Brownstein CA, Adler F, Nelson-Williams C, Iijima J, Li P, Imura A, Nabeshima Y, Reyes-Mugica M, Carpenter TO, Lifton RP: A translocation causing increased alpha-Klotho level results in hypophosphatemic rickets and hyperparathyroidism. Proc Natl Acad Sci U S A 2008;105:3455–3460.

36 Hafner C, van Oers JM, Vogt T, Landthaler M, Stoehr R, Blaszyk H, Hofstaedter F, Zwarthoff EC, Hartmann A: Mosaicism of activating FGFR3 mutations in human skin causes epidermal nevi. J Clin Invest 2006;116:2201–2207.

37 White KE, Cabral JM, Davis SI, Fishburn T, Evans WE, Ichikawa S, Fields J, Yu X, Shaw NJ, McLellan NJ, McKeown C, Fitzpatrick D, Yu K, Ornitz DM, Econs MJ: Mutations that cause osteoglophonic dysplasia define novel roles for FGFR1 in bone elongation. Am J Hum Genet 2005;76:361–367.

38 Araya K, Fukumoto S, Backenroth R, Takeuchi Y, Nakayama K, Ito N, Yoshii N, Yamazaki Y, Yamashita T, Silver J, Igarashi T, Fujita T: A novel mutation in fibroblast growth factor 23 gene as a cause of tumoral calcinosis. J Clin Endocrinol Metab 2005; 90:5523–5527.

39 Garringer HJ, Fisher C, Larsson TE, Davis SI, Koller DL, Cullen MJ, Draman MS, Conlon N, Jain A, Fedarko NS, Dasgupta B, White KE: The role of mutant UDP-N-acetyl-alpha-D-galactosamine-polypeptide N-acetylgalactosaminyltransferase 3 in regulating serum intact fibroblast growth factor 23 and matrix extracellular phosphoglycoprotein in heritable tumoral calcinosis. J Clin Endocrinol Metab 2006;91:4037–4042.

Dr. Dov Tiosano
Pediatric Endocrinology, Meyer Children's Hospital, Rambam Medical Center
Rappaport Family Faculty of Medicine, Technion-Israel Institute of Technology
IL–30196 Haifa (Israel)
Tel. +972 4 8542955, E-Mail d_tiosano@rambam.health.gov.il

Camacho-Hübner C, Nilsson O, Sävendahl L (eds): Cartilage and Bone Development and Its Disorders.
Endocr Dev. Basel, Karger, 2011, vol 21, pp 78–84

Molecular Defects Causing Skeletal Dysplasias

Outi Mäkitie

Hospital for Children and Adolescents, Pediatric Endocrinology and Metabolic Bone Diseases,
Helsinki University Hospital and University of Helsinki, Helsinki, Finland

Abstract

Almost 400 different forms of skeletal dysplasias have been described, each with characteristic clinical and radiographic features. The underlying genetic and molecular pathology is known in several forms. Correct diagnosis is important for genetic counseling, treatment decisions, follow-up and for predicting long-term outcome. With advances in molecular genetics it has become evident that variable phenotypes can be caused by mutations in one gene, depending on the mutation type and location within the gene. On the other hand, mutations in different genes can result in similar phenotypes. Careful clinical assessment with thorough radiographic evaluation are of key importance.

Skeletal Dysplasias

Skeletal development is regulated by numerous genetic factors that are only partly known. Accordingly, genetic disorders affecting the skeleton, or skeletal dysplasias, resulting from defects in these genes, comprise a large group of clinically distinct and genetically heterogeneous conditions. They are characterized by abnormalities in patterning, linear growth, differentiation, and maintenance of the human skeleton, beginning during fetal development and evolving throughout life. Clinical manifestations range from neonatal lethality to only mild growth retardation or deformity. Several skeletal dysplasias present prenatally or in early infancy with severe deformities and dwarfism. However, some forms are milder and present later in childhood with mild growth retardation or with unspecific skeletal symptoms. In such a situation, the diagnosis of skeletal dysplasia may be more challenging, especially if the presenting symptoms are not clearly confined to the skeleton.

More than 370 different forms of skeletal dysplasia have been described to date, each with a characteristic clinical and radiological presentation [1]. In several of these, the genetic basis of the disorder has been described and mutations in the responsible genes identified. Although they are individually rare, disorders of the skeleton are of clinical relevance because of their overall frequency. A correct diagnosis of the skeletal dysplasia has significant implications in genetic counseling when determining the mode of inheritance and the recurrence risk in affected families. Furthermore, a specific diagnosis is helpful in the follow-up and treatment of the patient and in predicting long-term outcome of the disorder.

Classification of Skeletal Dysplasias

Due to their clinical diversity, skeletal dysplasias are often difficult to diagnose, and many attempts have been made to delineate single entities or groups of diseases to facilitate diagnosis and to guide in clinical management of the patients.

The classification of the skeletal dysplasias was first limited to clinical and radiographic criteria. The resulting subgroups – e.g. metaphyseal, epiphyseal, spondylo-epiphyseal, and spondylo-epi-metaphyseal dysplasia – still include several different forms of skeletal dysplasia, but the subgrouping is helpful in further trying to identify the specific diagnosis and the underlying genetic pathology of the condition: determining the components of the skeleton that are abnormal in size, shape, and mineralization pattern is important in refining the differential diagnoses (fig. 1).

Kornak and Mundlos [2] suggested an alternative classification based on a combination of molecular pathology and embryology. They subdivided skeletal disorders into four major groups: (1) disorders affecting skeletal patterning (e.g. rib and vertebral malformations, polydactyly, absence defects of the limbs); (2) disorders affecting condensation/differentiation of skeletal precursor structures ('anlagen'; e.g. brachydactyly, defects of joint formation); (3) disorders of growth (e.g. impaired chondrocyte proliferation in metaphyseal chondrodysplasias, impaired bone matrix production in type II collagenopathies and osteogenesis imperfecta), and (4) disorders of skeletal homeostasis (e.g. disorders with abnormal bone mineralization or osteoblast function).

The most recent classification incorporates clinical, radiographic, and molecular features. In the 2006 revision of the International Nosology and Classification of Genetic Skeletal Disorders, 372 different conditions have been listed in 37 groups defined by molecular, biochemical, and/or radiographic criteria [1] (table 1).

It is apparent that no single classification of skeletal dysplasias will be adequate for diagnostic, clinical and research purposes, and novel classifications will probably be developed and refined as new clinical, radiographic, morphologic, biochemical, molecular, and pathway data emerge.

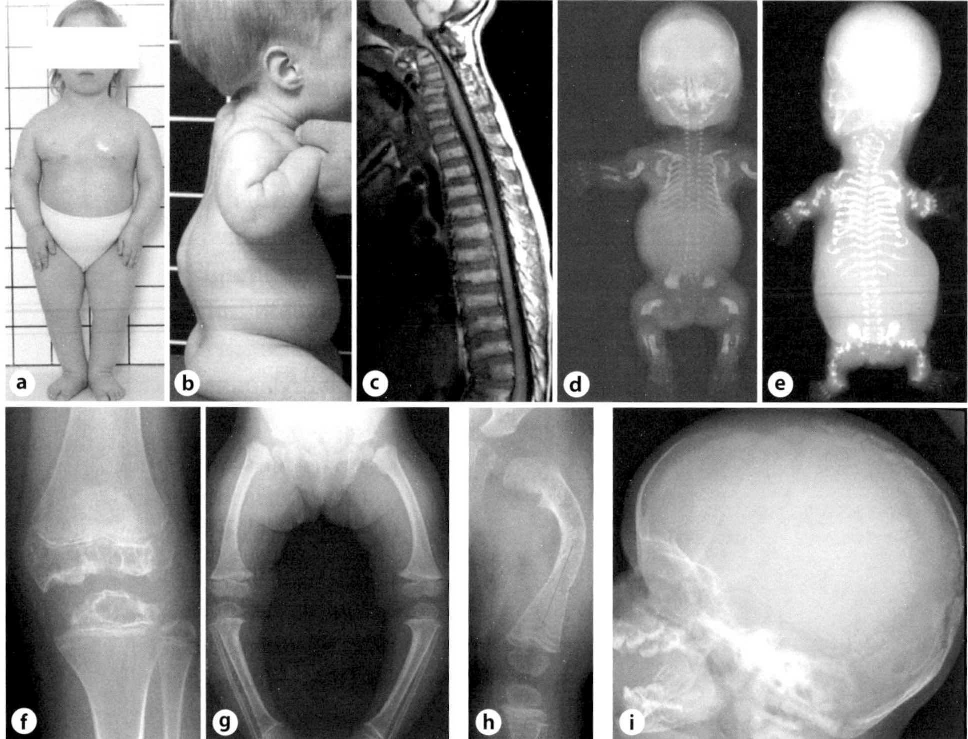

Fig. 1. Examples of skeletal dysplasias. **a** A 10-year-old child with cartilage-hair hypoplasia (height 87 cm). **b** Short stature, macrocephaly and lumbar kyphosis in a child with achondroplasia. **c** Vertebral abnormalities in a boy with spondylo-epiphyseal dysplasia. **d, e** Fetuses with lethal skeletal dysplasia. **f** Abnormal knee epiphysis in MED. **g** Radiographic findings of metaphyseal chondrodysplasia type Schmid. **h** Femoral bowing in an infant with severe osteogenesis imperfecta. **i** Cranial mineralization defect in cleidocranial dysplasia.

Skeletal Dysplasia Families

One Gene – Several Phenotypes

Achondroplasia is the most common non-lethal skeletal dysplasia and often regarded as the 'prototype' of skeletal dysplasias [3]. It is an autosomal dominant condition with an incidence between 1:10,000–1:30,000. The phenotype is characterized by disproportionate short stature with short limbs and long spine, enlarged head with frontal bossing and midface hypoplasia, short hands, lumbar lordosis, and normal cognitive functions. Achondroplasia is caused by a gain-of-function mutation in the gene encoding the FGFR3; in more than 95% of cases achondroplasia is caused by an identical missense mutation Gly380Arg in the transmembrane domain of FGFR3. Most of the mutations arise de novo. The clinical features and radiographic skeletal findings are essential in the diagnosis, and mutational analysis of *FGFR3* can be used to confirm the diagnosis.

Table 1. International nosology and classification of genetic skeletal disorders divide the skeletal dysplasias into 37 groups based on clinical, radiographic and molecular features, and examples of the groups of disorders are given

Group/specific diagnosis	Gene
FGFR3 group	
Thanatophoric dysplasia types 1 and 2	*FGFR3*
SADDAN (severe achondroplasia-developmental delay-acanthosis nigricans)	*FGFR3*
Achondroplasia	*FGFR3*
Hypochondroplasia	*FGFR3*
Type 2 collagen group	
Achondrogenesis type 2	*COL2A1*
Platyspondylic dysplasia, Torrance type	*COL2A1*
Hypochondrogenesis	*COL2A1*
Spondyloepiphyseal dysplasia congenital	*COL2A1*
Spondyloepimetaphyseal dysplasia	*COL2A1*
Kniest dysplasia	*COL2A1*
Spondyloepiphyseal dysplasia	*COL2A1*
Stickler syndrome type 1	*COL2A1*
Sulfation disorders group	
Achondrogenesis type 1B	*SLC26A2*
Atelosteogenesis type 2	*SLC26A2*
Diastrophic dysplasia	*SLC26A2*
MED, autosomal recessive	*SLC26A2*
Metaphyseal dysplasias	
Metaphyseal dysplasia, Schmid type	*COL10A1*
Cartilage-hair hypoplasia	*RMRP*
Metaphyseal dysplasia, Jansen type	*PTHR1*
Shwachman-Diamond syndrome	*SBDS*
Metaphyseal anadysplasia	*MMP13*
Metaphyseal dysplasia, Spahr type	

Interestingly, mutations in other parts of the *FGFR3* gene are associated with different skeletal dysplasias (table 1) [4]. Hypochondroplasia, characterized by a milder clinical and radiological phenotype, is caused by mutations in the tyrosine kinase domains 1 (Asn540Lys) and 2 (Lys650Glu or Lys650Asn) of the *FGFR3* gene, but also several other mutations in the *FGFR3* gene have been described [5]. Further, thanatophoric dwarfism, a neonatal lethal chondrodysplasia with severe shortening of the limbs with macrocephaly, narrow thorax and short ribs is caused by mutations in the extracellular domain of the same protein.

Diastrophic dysplasia is the most prevalent skeletal dysplasia in Finland; more than 180 Finnish patients are known. The clinical characteristics include short-limbed disproportionate short stature (adult height 95–140 cm) with associated joint dislocations, joint contractures, scoliosis and cleft palate. Diastrophic dysplasia is autosomal recessive and caused by bi-allelic mutations in the gene encoding a sulfate transporter protein that is essential for normal cartilage function [6]. Mutations in this *SLC26A2* gene cause diastrophic dysplasia but also atelosteogenesis type 2, a neonatal lethal chondrodysplasia, and a much milder skeletal dysplasia, the rMED. The severity of the phenotype depends on the degree of functional impairment of the sulphate transporter caused by the mutations [7].

Similar to achondroplasia and diastrophic dysplasia, several other 'dysplasia families' with similar genetic background (causative mutations in the same gene) but different phenotypic features have been identified. Some examples are summarized in table 1. As the phenotypic spectrum ranges from neonatal lethality to only mild skeletal impairment, not only the gene mutation but also its functional consequences have to be taken into account.

One Phenotype – Several Genes

On the other hand, it has been recognized that mutations in several genes may lie behind a particular phenotype. MED is an example of such a condition. It is a skeletal dysplasia characterized by joint pain and stiffness, waddling gait and/or mild short stature in childhood. Radiographic findings include abnormal development of epiphyses in multiple joints. The disorder is genetically heterogeneous [8]. Mutations in the *COMP* gene cause a dominantly inherited form of MED. However, mutations in the genes coding for the type IX collagen α-chains *(COL9A1*, *COL9A2* or *COL9A3)*, as well as mutations in the *MATN3* gene, encoding an extracellular matrix protein matrilin 3, also cause an autosomal dominant form of MED. In addition to these 5 dominant forms, rMED has also been described in which homozygous or compound heterozygous mutations in the sulphate transporter gene, *SLC26A2*, cause the phenotype [8].

Careful clinical and radiographic characterization of the MED patients may give hints regarding the genetic background [9]. Patients with *COMP* mutations usually have the most severe changes in the hip joints and a progressive disease leading to early-onset hip osteoarthritis, requiring joint replacement. In contrast, patients with collagen IX mutations typically have relative sparing of the hip joints, while the most drastic radiographic findings are observed in the knees. The hips and knees are the most commonly affected joints in patients with *MATN3* mutations, but the hip involvement is intermediate as compared with that caused by *COMP* or collagen IX mutations. The presence of epiphyseal changes in combination with a double-layered patella and/or clubfoot is characteristic of rMED caused by *SLC26A2* mutations.

Diagnosis

It is important to differentiate between the specific conditions for accurate genetic counseling, prognosis and treatment. Careful clinical examination, detailed radiographic evaluation of the skeleton and a multidisciplinary approach are needed when evaluating patients with chondrodysplasias. Since the genetic background of several skeletal dysplasias is known, molecular diagnostic tests should be utilized whenever possible. However, in clinical practice this may be challenging. As discussed previously, mutations in several genes may result in an identical phenotype and molecular genetic confirmation would require screening of several genes. For example, the MEDs include both dominant and recessive forms, and confirmation of the genetic defect behind the condition would be important for proper genetic counseling. However, in practice this is usually impossible due to the high number of genes to be screened and consequently the high cost of genetic testing. In order to avoid unnecessary tests, it is of utmost importance to appreciate the phenotypic findings and to use careful radiographic, biochemical and possibly histological approach in trying to establish the clinical diagnosis.

Many skeletal dysplasias present already during fetal development. Despite recent advances in imaging, fetal skeletal dysplasias are difficult to diagnose in utero due to the large number of skeletal dysplasias and their phenotypic variability and overlapping features, lack of precise molecular diagnosis for many disorders, and variability in the time at which findings manifest. Recent guidelines for prenatal diagnosis of fetal skeletal dysplasias [10] emphasize the importance of differentiating known lethal disorders from nonlethal disorders, providing differential diagnoses before delivery, determining postdelivery management plans and ultimately determining accurate diagnosis and recurrence risk.

Conclusions

During the past decade, enormous progress has been made in the understanding of the biochemical and molecular genetic basis of skeletal dysplasias. This enables the development of accurate diagnostic tests, but also provides broader insight into the pathogenesis, natural course and prognosis as well as potential therapeutic options for the specific conditions. There still remain a number of disorders in which the disease gene has not been identified. The cornerstone for a correct genetic diagnosis is reliable phenotypic delineation of the skeletal dysplasia in an affected individual. Preferably, the diagnostic workup, genetic counseling and clinical care of patients with skeletal dysplasia should be centralized to experienced multidisciplinary teams.

References

1 Superti-Furga A, Unger S: Nosology and classification of genetic skeletal disorders: 2006 revision. Am J Med Genet A 2007;143:1.

2 Kornak U, Mundlos S: Genetic disorders of the skeleton: a developmental approach. Am J Hum Genet 2003;73:447.

3 Horton WA, Hall JG, Hecht JT: Achondroplasia. Lancet 2007;370:162.

4 Vajo Z, Francomano CA, Wilkin DJ: The molecular and genetic basis of fibroblast growth factor receptor 3 disorders: the achondroplasia family of skeletal dysplasias, Muenke craniosynostosis, and Crouzon syndrome with acanthosis nigricans. Endocr Rev 2000;21:23.

5 Bellus GA, McIntosh I, Smith EA, Aylsworth AS, Kaitila I, Horton WA, Greenhaw GA, Hecht JT, Francomano CA: A recurrent mutation in the tyrosine kinase domain of fibroblast growth factor receptor 3 causes hypochondroplasia. Nat Genet 1995;10:357.

6 Rossi A, Superti-Furga A: Mutations in the diastrophic dysplasia sulfate transporter (DTDST) gene (SLC26A2): 22 novel mutations, mutation review, associated skeletal phenotypes, and diagnostic relevance. Hum Mutat 2001;17:159.

7 Karniski LP: Mutations in the diastrophic dysplasia sulfate transporter (DTDST) gene: correlation between sulfate transport activity and chondrodysplasia phenotype. Hum Mol Genet 2001;10:1485.

8 Jakkula E, Mäkitie O, Czarny-Ratajczak M, Jackson GC, Damignani R, Susic M, Briggs MD, Cole WG, Ala-Kokko L: Mutations in the known genes are not the major cause of MED; distinctive phenotypic entities among patients with no identified mutations. Eur J Hum Genet 2005;13:292.

9 Unger SL, Briggs MD, Holden P, Zabel B, Ala-Kokko L, Paassilta P, Lohiniva J, Rimoin DL, Lachman RS, Cohn DH: Multiple epiphyseal dysplasia: radiographic abnormalities correlated with genotype. Pediatr Radiol 2001;31:10.

10 Krakow D, Lachman RS, Rimoin DL: Guidelines for the prenatal diagnosis of fetal skeletal dysplasias. Genet Med 2009;11:127.

Dr. Outi Mäkitie
Hospital for Children and Adolescents, Pediatric Endocrinology and Metabolic Bone Diseases, Helsinki University Hospital and University of Helsinki
PO Box 281
FI–00029 HUS, Helsinki (Finland)
Tel. +358 44 2050155, E-Mail outi.makitie@helsinki.fi

Camacho-Hübner C, Nilsson O, Sävendahl L (eds): Cartilage and Bone Development and Its Disorders.
Endocr Dev. Basel, Karger, 2011, vol 21, pp 85–90

Allele-Specific Gene Silencing in Osteogenesis Imperfecta

Östen Ljunggren · Katarina Lindahl · Carl-Johan Rubin · Andreas Kindmark

Department of Medical Sciences, Uppsala University, Uppsala, Sweden

Abstract

OI is caused by mutations in the genes encoding for collagen type I *COL1A1* and *COL1A2*, respectively. The patients suffer from bone fragility, and the severity can range from mild, with fractures in the youth, to lethal forms. Today, there is no effective treatment for the disorder. OI is caused by dominant negative mutations. A tempting approach to treat the disease would be to silence the allele carrying the mutation. This could in theory be done with siRNAs. Today, more than 800 various mutations are reported, and to create siRNA against a specific mutation is difficult. Instead, by developing siRNA against common polymorphic variations, it would be possible to silence the mutation by a standardized method regardless where the mutation is located on the allele. If the concept of allele-specific gene silencing by inhibitory RNA directed towards dominant negative mutations could be proven, this might be a novel approach to gene therapy in OI.

Osteogenesis Imperfecta: Cause of Disease and Clinical Manifestations

OI is a heterogeneous genetic disorder with a prevalence of 1/10,000 to 1/15,000 individuals. The disease leads to an increased susceptibility to fracture. Classically, OI is divided into four subtypes, Sillence classification I–IV, with the addition of three more rare forms. Type I is the most common form and is generally mild and non-deforming [1]. Patients reach near normal stature and have average life span expectancy. Type II is the most severe and is lethal already in the perinatal period, usually due to respiratory insufficiency from multiple thoracic fractures. Type III is severely deforming, and patients often have fractures at birth. Type IV has a clinical range between type I and III, and thus is moderately deforming. Recently described types V–VII are rare and lead to a moderate to severe phenotype [2, 3].

In more than 90% of patients with OI type I–IV, the disorder is due to a dominant mutation in one of the two genes that encode the α-chains of collagen type I, Col1A1 and Col1A2 [4]. Collagen I is present in many tissues, and in addition to multiple fractures, patients with OI can have dentinogenesis imperfecta, blue sclera, hypermobile ligaments and skin, hearing loss and increased risk of bruising. The majority of patients with OI have a low bone mineral density [5].

Collagen type I is synthesized as a soluble precursor, procollagen, that is made up of two chains of proα1 and one chain of proα2 propeptides. Both proα1 and proα2 have a central region of about 1,000 amino acids with a glycine at every third position that, with the help of a C-terminal globular region, creates a triple helix terminated by an N-terminal globular region. Glycine is the only amino acid small enough to fit in the middle of the tightly packed helix, and is therefore a prerequisite for correct folding and helix formation. Once out of the cell, procollagen will be cleaved enzymatically and lose its globular ends, and the remaining triple helix will assemble into fibrils automatically. This organic frame can subsequently be mineralized by hydroxyapatite.

There are more than 800 different mutations reported with an OI phenotype as outcome [5]. Type I OI is usually the result of a mutation that leads to a premature stop codon, which in turn leads to too little, but structurally normal collagen. This type of mutation is usually clustered in families. In contrast, the more severe OI phenotypes are often de-novo mutations which lead to an exchange of a glycine residue in the triple helix for an amino acid with a bulkier side chain. Other known mutations lead to exon skipping and changed splice sites. Rare mutations have been reported in the N- and C-terminal portions of the propeptide [6].

To date there is no cure for OI. Many patients are treated with bisphosphonates, but only for some is there support from data obtained in clinical trials [7]. However, little is known about which patients benefit from this treatment and which do not. It is not known if treatment with other osteoporosis drugs would be a better alternative or perhaps a complement to bisphosphonates in treating patients with OI.

Current Treatment Options

There is currently no effective treatment for OI. Most patients are still treated with orthopedic surgery, rehabilitation and physiotherapy. Bisphosphonates are the drug of choice for symptomatic treatment of patients with OI [8], but their effect is neither sufficient nor satisfactory. Treatment with other osteoporosis drugs, such as anabolic treatment with teriparatide could be a more beneficial alternative or perhaps a complement to bisphosphonate treatment in patients with OI. The knowledge of which patients would benefit from certain treatment regimes is limited as treatment efficacy may be in part related to the type of mutation.

Stem Cell Transfer

Studies of individuals being mosaic carriers of OI-causing mutations [9, 10] and bone marrow transplantation as investigational treatment in patients with OI and studies of murine OI models have shown that even a very small increase in cells producing normal collagen can have a striking effect on bone phenotype [11–13]. This is encouraging not only for stem cell transfer as a future treatment modality, but also for the gene silencing approach as only a slight shift towards normalization might carry a significant clinical effect.

Gene Silencing by Inhibitory RNA

A therapeutic vision is to convert a severe OI type to a type I OI by silencing the mutated gene. One possible approach would be to use gene silencing through RNAi. The attractiveness of RNAi in contrast to other molecular methods arises from its high inhibitory activity and the fact that the inhibition is very specific [14, 15]. RNAi is the process by which cellular RNA is targeted for degradation upon exposure to complementary RNA. In 1999, siRNAs were discovered as endogenous molecules mediating RNAi in plants [16], and in 2001 it was shown that exogenous double-stranded siRNAs efficiently reduced mRNA levels in animal cells in vitro [17]. Since these seminal discoveries, the siRNA technology has been further developed, and siRNAs are now invaluable tools for studies of partial gene knockout in vitro as well as in vivo [18]. Recent studies have reported successful allele-specific gene silencing by siRNAs that discriminate between single nucleotide variants within mRNAs [19–21]. These studies suggest that siRNAs may be interesting to explore as therapeutics in monogenic disorders where the dysfunctional allele could be targeted specifically.

More than 800 mutations causing OI through structural collagen changes have been described in *COL1A1* and *COL1A2* [5], and new mutations are frequently reported. Hence, the need is for creating a large number of unique siRNAs, each targeting one single mutation. This would be extremely labor intensive. An alternative is to use a mutation-independent approach, designing siRNAs that target common *COL1A1* and *COL1A2* SNPs [22, 23]. However, satisfactory allele specificity may prove difficult to achieve considering that the two alleles differ by only one nucleotide in a heterozygous individual. Therefore, a theoretically attractive approach is to use siRNAs targeting heterozygotes for insertions/deletions. In this case, the two alleles differ by more than one nucleotide, which should increase the chance of true allele specificity.

The actual delivery of siRNAs is another hurdle, but recent advances in adenoviral vector-based gene therapy are compliant with siRNAs and have been used for cell type-specific siRNA expression, as have other approaches in vivo in murine models

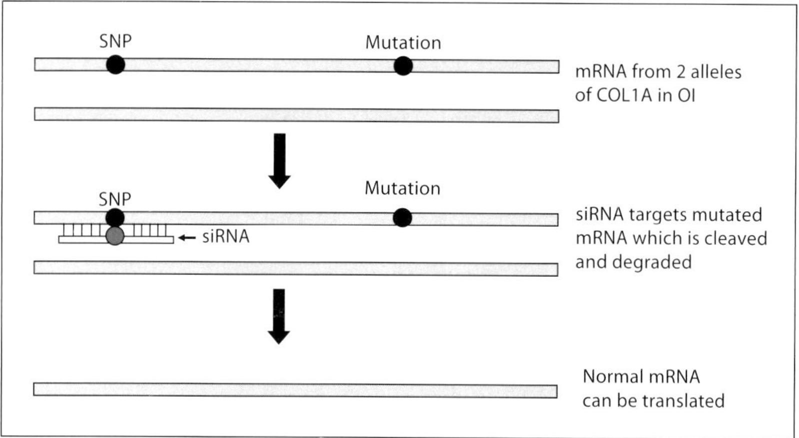

Fig. 1. Allele-specific silencing of a mutated gene by using common polymorphic variations as target. OI is caused by dominant negative mutations. Today, more than 800 various mutations are reported, and to create siRNA against a specific mutation is difficult. Instead, by developing siRNA against common polymorphic variations it would be possible to silence the mutation by a standardized method regardless where the mutation is located on the allele.

[24]. Furthermore, there is a rapid development in the clinic using various vectors to deliver siRNA in a variety of disorders [25]. However, these are all diseases where complete silencing of a gene is of benefit. Therefore, it is easy to construct a siRNA that can suppress both alleles. In the case of dominant negative disorders, such as OI, the task is much more difficult since only one allele is to be targeted. Recently, however, we published the first evidence that this might be possible in OI showing data on allele-specific silencing in vitro by using tiling siRNAs against polymorphic variations in one collagen allele (fig. 1) [23].

Future Challenges Regarding siRNAs in Osteogenesis Imperfecta

Although promising, several obstacles must be overcome before truly allele-specific siRNAs that render 50% silencing of *COL1A1* or *COL1A2* can be tested in clinical trials. SiRNA sequences will need to be optimized to achieve maximum efficiency and specificity as the base composition is of utmost importance for RNAi outcome. Furthermore, siRNAs are likely to contain sequences partially complementary to other genes, which necessitates excluding undesirable and potentially deleterious off target effects. An appropriate vehicle for delivery of the siRNAs in vitro and eventually in vivo will be essential, and it will also be necessary to determine how to administer siRNAs specifically to the target cells in sufficient quantity.

Conclusions

OI is caused by mutations in the genes encoding for collagen type I. The patients suffer from multiple fractures, and at the moment there is no curative treatment. Bisphosphonates are used with some effect, but in order to treat the most severe cases either stem cell transfer or gene silencing are suggested as treatment. The field of siRNA is advancing fast as a potential treatment for a variety of diseases believed to benefit from gene silencing. In OI, this therapeutic approach requires allele-specific silencing which poses the hurdle of specificity. The finding that allele-specific silencing of collagen alleles is possible in vitro [23] in human bone-derived cell using siRNAs targeting common polymorphisms suggests a novel approach towards personalized RNAi therapy in severe OI.

Acknowledgement

We thank technicians and study nurses at the Uppsala Osteoporosis Research Unit for skilful assistance. This work was supported by grants from the Swedish Research Council, project No. 2007-2946.

References

1 Sillence DO, Rimoin DL, Danks DM: Clinical variability in osteogenesis imperfecta-variable expressivity or genetic heterogeneity. Birth Defects Orig Artic Ser 1979;15:13.

2 Ward LM, Rauch F, Travers R, Chabot G, Azouz EM, Lalic L, Roughley PJ, Glorieux FH: Osteogenesis imperfecta type VII: an autosomal recessive form of brittle bone disease. Bone 2002;31:12.

3 Glorieux FH, Ward LM, Rauch F, Lalic L, Roughley PJ, Travers R: Osteogenesis imperfecta type VI: a form of brittle bone disease with a mineralization defect. J Bone Miner Res 2002;1:30.

4 Byers PH, Wallis GA, Willing MC: Osteogenesis imperfecta, translation of genotype to phenotype. J Med Genet 1991;28:433.

5 Marini JC, Forlino A, Cabral WA, et al: Consortium for osteogenesis imperfecta mutations in the helical domain of type I collagen: regions rich in lethal mutations align with collagen binding sites for integrins and proteoglycans. Hum Mutat 2007;28:209.

6 Rauch F, Glorieux FH: Bisphosphonate treatment in osteogenesis imperfecta: which drug, for whom, for how long? Ann Med 2005;37:295.

7 Phillini CA, Remmington T, Steiner RD: Bisphosphonate therapy for osteogenesis imperfecta. Cochrane Database Syst Rev 2008;CD005088.

8 Castillo H, Samson-Fang L: Effects of bisphosphonates in children with osteogenesis imperfecta: an AACPDM systematic review. Dev Med Child Neurol 2009;51:17.

9 Raghunath M, Mackay K, Dalgleish R, Steinmann B: Genetic counselling on brittle grounds: recurring osteogenesis imperfecta due to parental mosaicism for a dominant mutation. Eur J Pediatr 1995; 154:123.

10 Cabral WA, Marini JC: High proportion of mutant osteoblasts is compatible with normal skeletal function in mosaic carriers of osteogenesis imperfecta. Am J Hum Genet 2004;74:752.

11 Horwitz EM, Prockop DJ, Gordon PL, Koo WW, Fitzpatrick LA, Neel MD, McCarville ME, Orchard PJ, Pyeritz RE, Brenner MK: Clinical responses to bone marrow transplantation in children with severe osteogenesis imperfecta. Blood 2001;97: 1227.

12 Horwitz EM, Gordon PL, Koo WK, Marx JC, Neel MD, McNall RY, Muul L, Hofmann T: Isolated allogeneic bone marrow-derived mesenchymal cells engraft and stimulate growth in children with osteogenesis imperfecta: implications for cell therapy of bone. Proc Natl Acad Sci USA 2002;99:8932.

13 Panaroni C, Gioia R, Lupi A, Besio R, Goldstein SA, Kreider J, Leikin S, Vera JC, Mertz EL, Perilli E, Baruffaldi F, Villa I, Farina A, Casasco M, Cetta G, Rossi A, Frattini A, Marini JC, Vezzoni P, Forlino A: In utero transplantation of adult bone marrow decreases perinatal lethality and rescues the bone phenotype in the knockin murine model for classical, dominant osteogenesis imperfecta. Blood 2009;114:459.

14 Miller VM, Xia H, Marrs GL, Gouvion CM, Lee G, Davidson BL, Paulson HL: Allele-specific silencing of dominant disease genes. Proc Natl Acad Sci USA 2003;100:7195.

15 Abdelgany A, Wood M, Beeson D: Allele-specific silencing of a pathogenic mutant acetylcholine receptor subunit by RNA interference. Hum Mol Genet 2003;12:2637.

16 Hamilton AJ, Baulcombe DC: A species of small antisense RNA in posttranscriptional gene silencing in plants. Science 1999;286:950.

17 Elbashir SM, Harborth J, Lendeckel W, Yalcin A, Weber K, Tuschl T: Duplexes of 21-nucleotide RNAs mediate RNA interference in cultured mammalian cells. Nature 2001;411:494.

18 Zimmermann TS, Lee AC, Akinc A, et al: RNAi-mediated gene silencing in non-human primates. Nature 2006;441:111.

19 Dykxhoorn DM, Schlehuber LD, London I M, Lieberman J: Determinants of specific RNA interference-mediated silencing of human beta-globin alleles differing by a single nucleotide polymorphism. Proc Natl Acad Sci USA 2006;103:5953.

20 Hickerson R P, Smith FJ, Reeves RE, Contag CH, Leake D, Leachman SA, Milstone LM, McLean WH, Kaspar RL: Single-nucleotide-specific siRNA targeting in a dominant-negative skin model. J Invest Dermatol 2008;128:594.

21 Schwarz DS, Ding H, Kennington L, Moore JT, Schelter J, Burchard J, Linsley PS, Aronin N, Xu Z, Zamore PD: Designing siRNA that distinguish between genes that differ by a single nucleotide. PLoS Genet 2006;2:e140.

22 Millington-Ward S, McMahon H P, Allen D, Tuohy G, Kiang AS, Palfi A, Kenna PF, Humphries P, Farrar GJ: RNAi of COL1A1 in mesenchymal progenitor cells. Eur J Hum Genet 2004;12:864.

23 Lindahl K, Rubin CJ, Kindmark A, Ljunggren Ö: Allele dependent silencing of COL1A2 using small interfering RNAs. Int J Med Sci 2008;5:361.

24 McNamara JO 2nd, Andrechek ER, Wang Y, Viles KD, Rempel RE, Gilboa E, Sullenger BA, Giangrande PH: Cell type-specific delivery of siRNAs with aptamersiRNA chimeras. Nat Biotechnol 2006;24:1005.

25 Whitehead KA Langer R, Anderson DG: Knocking down barriers: advances in siRNA delivery. Nat Rev 2009;8:129–138.

Prof. Östen Ljunggren
Department of Medical Sciences, Uppsala University
SE–751 85 Uppsala (Sweden)
Tel. +46 18 611 0000, E-Mail Osten.ljunggren@medsci.uu.se

Camacho-Hübner C, Nilsson O, Sävendahl L (eds): Cartilage and Bone Development and Its Disorders.
Endocr Dev. Basel, Karger, 2011, vol 21, pp 91–101

Stem Cells in Skeletal Physiology and Endocrine Diseases of Bone

Paolo Bianco · Benedetto Sacchetti · Mara Riminucci

Department of Molecular Medicine, La Sapienza University, and Biomedical Science Park San Raffaele, Rome, Italy

Abstract

Self-renewing, multipotent progenitors of skeletal tissues are found within skeletal segments (skeletal stem cells) and coincide with adventitial reticular cells of bone marrow vessels in situ and with explanted clonogenic stromal cells ex vivo. These cells, which can be identified and prospectively isolated based on a minimal surface phenotype noted for expression of CD146, CD105 and alkaline phosphatase, are established during bone development through interactions with developing sinusoids. They represent a crucial crossroad of skeletal and hematopoietic physiology, as well as of endocrine regulation of bone growth and remodeling. In addition, they are central to major endocrine functions of bone itself, such as regulation of renal phosphate handling. Skeletal stem cells represent a central model system for investigating skeletal diseases, as tools for in vitro and in vivo models, for cell therapy-based strategies, or as targets for drugs.

Skeletal Stem Cells

The view of the skeleton as a system of tissues rooted into a common ancestor that can be identified within the bone marrow originates from classical experiments going back at least to the 1960s. It was through heterotopic transplantation of boneless bone marrow fragments that the existence of an osteogenic potential was first identified [1]. Later, major refinements of the same fundamental experimental approach led to assigning this osteogenic potential to the nonhematopoietic (stromal) component of the bone marrow, and then to single cells, noted for an inherent capacity to generate clonal colonies in culture, and endowed with obvious multipotency [2–7]. Upon proper in vivo assays, these cells were in fact capable of generating histology-proven bone, cartilage, adipocytes, and fibrous tissue, thus highlighting the existence of a common multipotent progenitor for four distinct tissues found within individual skeletal segments (bone, cartilage, fibrous tissue and marrow adipocytes). From these data, the concept of an 'osteogenic' [8], or 'stromal' [9] stem cell was formulated to denote a putative second type of stem cell within the bone marrow, besides the hematopoietic stem cell. For a long time, two questions remained unaddressed: (1) whether the multipotent progenitor capable of initiating clonal growth would also be capable of self-renewal, the defining property of stem cells at large, and (2) whether the putative stromal stem cells could be identified with any more precision than allowed by classical cell biology studies, and traced to a recognizable cell type within the bone marrow stroma in situ.

Adventitial Cells as Skeletal Stem Cells

The paradigm for this kind of studies is provided by the success story of the identification of the murine hematopoietic stem cells [10, 11]. By seeking a phenotype for HSCs that would be based on surface antigens, it was possible to prospectively isolate, purify, and serially transplant mouse HSCs, proving their ability to reconstitute hematopoiesis in vivo at the single cell level, as well as their ability to self-renew, as illustrated by serial hematopoietic reconstitution in the mouse. For a long time, the lack of markers suited to identify the putative skeletal stem cell prevented progress in their identification beyond the notion that they would be stromal cells and would be comprised within the clonogenic subset thereof. Initial attempts to identify surface epitopes expressed in clonogenic stromal cells led to major advances in our ability to enrich, or nearly purify, the clonogenic subset, noted for high expression of a glycolipid surface epitope recognized by the Stro-1 antibody [12]. The characteristics of the Stro-1 antibody, however, prevented the identification of the clonogenic, Stro-1-expressing cells in situ. Through the use of different antigens that are coexpressed with Stro-1 in explanted stromal cells, but can also be identified by immunolabeling in situ, we now know that explanted, clonogenic stromal cells are noted for expression of CD146 (fig. 1), CD105, and with variable frequency alkaline phosphatase, and that coexpression of these antigens is seen, in vivo, in adventitial stromal cells of the bone marrow microvasculature [13], which appear to correspond to the adventitial reticular cells of classical histology [14–16].

Availability of antibodies to CD146/MCAM [17] that recognize the relevant epitope in decalcified paraffin-embedded material then allowed to correlate ex vivo studies (i.e. identification of the phenotype of the clonogenic stromal progenitors) not only with characterization of stromal cells in situ, but also with following their fate through culture and after in vivo transplantation. This led to the observation that once prospectively isolated as $CD146^{hi}$ clonogenic cells, $CD146^{hi}$ adventitial stromal cells generate a clonal progeny in culture, which retains high and homogeneous expression of the same antigen. Upon in vivo transplantation along with an osteoconductive carrier in an open transplantation system, this progeny generates bone-forming osteoblasts, hematopoiesis-supporting stroma, and adipocytes. At the same

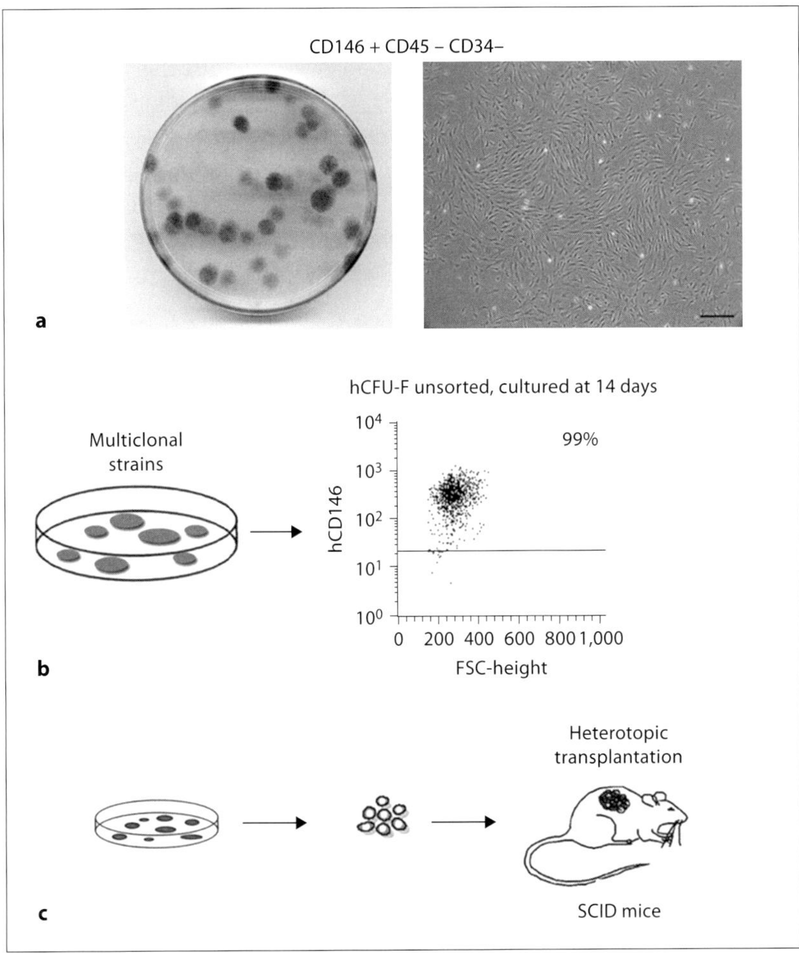

Fig. 1. a Isolation of skeletal stem cells. Skeletal stem cells can be prospectively isolated based on expression of CD146 at high levels in the CD34– CD45– bone marrow fraction. Once plated in culture at clonal density, they generate discrete colonies each of which represents a clone (clonogenic stromal cells, colony-forming units-fibroblastic, CFU-Fs). Either the whole culture, or individual clones are then expanded to generate a multiclonal progeny or a clonal progeny. **b** FACS analysis of a single clone at 14 days reveals homogeneous expression of CD146; forward scatter (FSC). **c** Expanded progenies are assayed for differentiation by heterotopic transplantation in the immunocompromised mouse. When osteogenic potential is being assayed, cells are first combined with an osteoconductive scaffold, typically consisting of a mixture of hydroxyapatite and tricalcium phosphate. Histology-proven human bone and bone marrow stroma form in 2 months in vivo, and are colonized by host hematopoietic cells.

time, a subset of CD146-expressing cells dynamically associates with developing sinusoids within the heterotopic ossicle, and self-renews into cells identical to adventitial reticular cells in the human bone marrow, i.e. to the cells originally explanted [13]. Importantly, the newly established adventitial stromal cells of heterotopic ossicles can be observed in secondary passages, demonstrating that assayable clonogenic cells can form from assayable clonogenic cells. These data provide evidence for the ability of $CD146^{hi}$, adventitial stromal cells, to self-renew in vivo, and thus establish these cells as bona fide stem cells [13, 18].

The Assayable Potency of Skeletal Stem Cells

The notion that bone marrow stromal cells could represent stem cells for a nonhematopoietic system of connective tissues found in the skeleton [8, 9] was reformulated in the late 1990s into a quite divergent concept that gained widespread popularity [19]. 'Mesenchymal stem cells' quickly became much more popular than 'osteogenic', stromal, or skeletal stem cells had ever been or would ever be as such. While 'MSCs' [20] originally coincided with the BM putative osteogenic stem cell of Friedenstein and others [8, 9], the concept of MSCs is quite distinct from that of skeletal stem cells, in three important respects. First, MSCs are widely thought to be endowed with a much broader differentiation potential than skeletal stem cells, including a number of extraskeletal and even nonmesoderm-derived lineages such as striated muscle, myocardium, endothelial cells, liver and neurons. Second, whereas skeletal stem cells are proven to exist within the skeleton, MSCs are thought to exist in virtually every organ [21]. Third, whereas the potency of skeletal stem cells is defined by stringent in vivo transplantation assays of clonal populations, the potency of MSCs is commonly assessed by artificial in vitro assays, most often conducted on nonclonal populations [reviewed in 18]. Whereas the skeletogenic potential of skeletal stem cells is solidly proven by in vivo transplantation data that have been reproduced in a number of laboratories worldwide, the nonskeletogenic potential of MSCs has not been proven with the same stringency or reproducibility, and current data seem to dispel at least the notion that MSCs can truly generate lineages distant from the skeletal phenotypes. When gauged through in vivo transplantation assays, skeletal stem cells derived from the adult bone marrow can differentiate into osteoblasts, marrow adipocytes, hematopoiesis-supporting stromal cells, adventitial reticular cells, and also into nondescript fibroblasts. They can establish the hematopoietic microenvironment at heterotopic sites, allowing for the appearance of hematopoietic niches within heterotopic ossicles. Although they cannot differentiate into endothelial cells [13], they can guide the formation of blood vessels and provide mural cells to the newly formed vessels [13]. Whether they can also generate cartilage in vivo is a somewhat controversial issue. Currently, in vitro micromass cell culture assays (so-called 'pellet assays') are employed to assess chondrogenic potential. In these systems, stromal cells can generate cartilage beads that sometimes fit the bill for histology-proven cartilage. Often, however, results of these assays are interpreted with an excess of optimism, but fall short of demonstrating true cartilage. In all cases, importantly, true or less convincing cartilage differentiation is induced ex vivo by exogenous cues conveying major reprogramming effects, such as those exerted by BMPs employed to doctor the putative stem cell into cartilage [reviewed in 22, 23]. Classical observations revealed that stromal cells from a number of species can indeed generate cartilage in diffusion chambers, in vivo and with no ex vivo induction. However, cartilage is not as easily formed in open transplantation systems in which blood vessels from the host can grow. This was originally, and still commonly is, interpreted in light of the low oxygen tension required for true cartilage differentiation, but alternative explanations exist. It is possible, for example, that chondrogenic potential may not be retained throughout life, and may be selectively lost at the end of skeletal growth. Further in vivo studies including comparative assessment of prenatal and postnatal bone marrow, as well as infantile vs. adult, are needed to elucidate this point.

Skeletal Stem Cells and the Hematopoietic Niche

The concept of skeletal stem cells has been intertwined with the concept of hematopoietic microenvironment/niche right from its very birth. Over more than 40 years, the use of entire bone marrow [1], stromal cell populations [24], single stromal clones [25, 26], and ultimately phenotype-purified stromal cells [13] in heterotopic transplantation systems marks the progressive refinement of the identification of skeletal progenitor cells that establish the hematopoietic microenvironment. It is now becoming apparent that the two systems of stem cells that reside in the bone marrow, actually reside in the same microvascular (sinusoidal) niche [13], and are likely engaged in substantial cross-regulation. This emerging view reconciles the two seemingly divergent notions that assign the hematopoietic stem cell niche either to osteoblasts [27, 28] (residing over endosteal surfaces) or to sinusoidal walls [29, for reviews see 30–32]. It is now clear that not only sinusoidal walls can be directly contiguous to endosteal surfaces, but sinusoidal walls include themselves osteogenic cells. The latter are not mature osteoblasts, but osteoblast progenitors residing, as adventitial reticular cells, next to the endothelial wall.

Skeletal Stem Cells and Bone Physiology

Traditionally centered on the paradigm of bone remodeling are two classes of mature cells, osteoblasts and osteoclasts; bone physiology finds in the notion of skeletal stem cells a true paradigm shift. As progenitors of osteoblasts, and as the provider of the specific cue to osteoclastogenesis, bone marrow stromal cells introduce cell proliferation and differentiation, rather than differentiated function, as a focus of studies centered on bone metabolism. As targets of major hormonal and local regulators of bone metabolism, bone marrow stromal cells also link cell growth and differentiation not only to differentiated cell function but also to general and local control of bone turnover. As mediators of the effects of disease-causing mutations, and possibly of the interaction of cancer with the bone environment, bone marrow stromal cells extend the range of skeletal diseases that can be profitably modeled through a cell biology approach [33]. Not surprisingly, culture systems based on isolation of stromal cells have become the dominant tool of such an approach. Nonetheless, progress in understanding bone physiology and disease through stem cells is a function of progress in understanding the nature and biology of the stem cells system under study, which in spite of some major progress and an unquestionable mass success, still remains in its infancy. Currently inscribed in a growing (exploding) attention to stem cell biology at large, the skeletal stem cell system is likely unique in many respects when compared with other stem cell systems. For example, renewal of the skeleton throughout the adult life is orders of magnitude slower than renewal of blood or epidermis [34], which implies that majorly different stem cell kinetics must operate in the different systems. Bone growth and adult remodeling are in and of themselves obviously distinct physiological processes, and may deserve specific consideration of relevant stem cell dynamics. For example, growth plates represent one of the clearest examples of self-renewing systems of progenitors [22], and yet they are by nature and definition transient, and thus defy the general (and yet, operational) definition of stem cell systems as lasting lifelong. Furthermore, little attention is paid to the circumstance that growth plates actually fuel the growth of the bone marrow cavity, rather than bone itself. Cortical bone grows longitudinally exactly at the same rate as the marrow cavity, but its growth is fueled by the periosteum. Whereas the resting zone of growth plates would be the natural niche for growth plate-fueling cartilage stem cells, how the longitudinal growth of bone cortices is maintained and actually strictly coordinated with the growth of the marrow cavity is largely unknown. The anatomic site where periosteal progenitors are retained during growth is likely to coincide with the time-honored Ranvier's groove [35], but studies directly targeting this forgotten anatomical structure are few and erratic.

Developmental Origin of Skeletal Stem Cells

As skeletal stem cells are found within the bone marrow, they are not established in development before the time when the bone marrow is established itself. This coincides with the cavity formation/vascular invasion phase of endochondral bone formation, which follows the establishment of the bony collar and therefore of the first osteoblasts. Paradoxically, the postnatal progenitors of osteoblasts arise in development after osteoblasts themselves have first appeared [36]. The growth of blood vessels from the primitive periosteum into the developing marrow cavity brings osteogenic progenitor cells from the periosteum into the developing cavity. This occurs prior to the remodeling of ingrowing blood vessels into sinusoids, which is followed by the immigration of blood-borne hematopoietic and progenitor cells. These seed the marrow cavity and establish contact with the extravascular stroma, resulting in the establishment of hematopoiesis. While this process first occurs in the center of the bone anlage, it then extends towards the proximal and distal epiphyses. In this way, the diaphyseal aspect of the growth plates becomes the site of transition between the primary spongiosa and the primitive marrow cavity. An extended view of the growth plates would thus include, next to the site of ossification, the site of bone marrow formation, as the leading edge of the expanding marrow cavity. The formation of the bone marrow cavity is altered in mice in which a constitutively active PTH/PTHrP receptor is expressed in osteoblasts [37], leading to a delayed formation of the marrow cavity due to an extended and protracted phase of bone formation at the diaphyseal aspect of the growth plates [38]. This suggests that PTH/PTHrP signaling modulates the formation of the marrow cavity through its own precisely timed regulation.

The establishment of the bone marrow and its stroma are recapitulated in in vivo transplantation systems using human skeletal stem cells. These systems typically employ mineral-based osteoconductive scaffolds such as hydroxyapatite/tricalcium phosphate mixtures [39], which functionally substitute for the mineralized cartilage scaffold seen in the natural growth plates. These scaffolds also feature an internal porosity, which is enhanced in their granular forms. They are efficiently resorbed by osteoclasts, like mineralized cartilage and bone. Following transplantation, bone is formed along the external and internal scaffold surfaces, followed by establishment of bone marrow only in the internal microcavities. As highlighted by transplantation systems, the establishment of skeletal stem cells in the newly developing hematopoietic cavities is inextricably linked with the formation of sinusoids and the recruitment of stromal cells to their outer wall [13]. Direct interaction of mesenchymal cells with endothelial cells triggers important regulatory events, mediated at least in part by TGF-β signaling and angiopoietin-1 [40, 41], which lead to the stabilization of both endothelial cells and the associated mesenchymal mural cells. The stabilization events induce mitotic quiescence and refractoriness to apoptosis in both endothelial cells and mural cells [42]. In this way, newly formed vessels are prevented from disappearing through microvascular pruning, while osteogenic cells are retained as mural cells (adventitial cells) around bone marrow sinusoids. Their primitive osteogenic nature is reflected in the constitutive expression of certain early osteogenic genes in bone marrow stromal cells, first and foremost the master gene of osteogenesis RUNX2 [43].

Skeletal Stem Cells and Skeletal Diseases

While there is currently a surge of interest in strategies for engineering bone tissues through skeletal stem cells, in various combinations with scaffolds of different chemical composition, physical structure, and biological activity [44], skeletal stem cells can enlighten understanding and treatment of bone diseases in at least three different, additional ways. First, they provide a system in which fundamental pathogenic events can be modeled, in a variety of diseases but most potently in monogenic diseases that affect bone. Second, they can provide a novel target for drugs. Third, they can provide a tool for strategies based on cell and gene therapy. Perhaps the single bone disease in which the significance of skeletal stem cells in these respects has been clearly highlighted is fibrous dysplasia of bone/McCune Albright syndrome (OMIM#174800) [45], a genetic disease caused by activating missense mutations of the GNAS gene, which encodes the α-subunit of the stimulatory G protein Gs. A crippling and rarely lethal disease arising in childhood or adolescence, FD is noted for a characteristic subversion of the architecture of the bone/bone marrow organ, with the focal loss of hematopoiesis and marrow adipocytes that are replaced by fibrosis, and the deposition of a structurally and functionally abnormal system of bone trabeculae [46, 47]. In vivo transplantation of Gsα-mutated stromal cells derived from FD lesions generates FD-like heterotopic ossicles, making a strong case for FD as a stromal cell disease [48, 49]. Subsequent use of FD-derived skeletal progenitors in both in vivo and in vitro studies has significantly contributed to our understanding of FD pathophysiology, highlighting for example the role of bone and osteogenic cells as producers of the phosphate-regulating hormone, FGF-23 [50], and thus disclosing a previously unrecognized nature of bone as an endocrine organ regulating phosphatemia. Analysis of the relative frequency of normal and mutated skeletal progenitors within FD lesions (the disease is a somatic mosaic, in which WT and mutated cells coexist) has also revealed that significant changes in stem cell kinetics are brought about by Gsα mutations that are reflected in defined patterns of evolution of the lesions itself over time and as a function of skeletal maturation [51]. More recently, the use of lentiviral technologies for stable transduction and gene silencing have allowed to generate strains of de novo mutated skeletal progenitors that are specifically suited to the study of downstream effects of the mutation, as matched to controls represented by the exact same strain of cells, untransduced. Initial characterization of these human transgenic stem cells has allowed to identify important effects of the mutation, such as the adaptive upregulation of certain phosphodiesterases, and the induction of a pro-osteoclastogenic signature centered on a reduced RANK-L/OPG ratio [52]. Importantly, RNA interference can be profitably coupled to lentiviral technologies to produce vectors that can stably silence individual genes. This theoretically provides a strategy for gene therapy in skeletal stem cells, followed by stem cell transplantation, a strategy made difficult by the current lack of effective ways to target the entire skeleton systemically. In FD specifically, additional complexity to gene therapy is added by the nature of the causative mutation, which is dominant and gain-of-function, and affects an indispensable ubiquitous gene. This leaves selective silencing of the mutated allele as the only conceivable strategy for gene therapy, a strategy made difficult in FD, again, by the circumstance that the causative mutation is a point mutation. While many barriers remain in the way to effective or even reasonable therapeutic trials, pursuing this avenue seems at least feasible or useful at this time. We have shown that lentivirus-directed RNAi is efficient in human skeletal progenitors, and can be specifically used to silence the FD mutation both in de novo transduced cells and in natural FD-derived progenitors [52]. The fundamental cellular phenotype induced by the mutation, i.e. the overproduction of cAMP due to Gsα overactivity, can be efficiently reverted through gene silencing. Furthermore, certain characteristic changes in the differentiation potential of Gsα-mutated skeletal progenitors, such as the loss of adipogenic differentiation, can in turn be reverted, at least in de novo transduced cells. Pursuing these studies will elucidate which mutation effects can be reverted, in what time, and to what extent, and might identify bottlenecks represented by cellular effects that in contrast cannot be easily reverted by normalizing Gsα function. Hence, a wealth of crucial information that can be translated into therapeutic strategies can be obtained along the way to gene therapy or stem cell therapy of bone disease, no matter how winding and steep the way.

Acknowledgments

Personal work cited in this article was supported in part by grants from Telethon GGP09227, MIUR, the EU and Fondazione Roma to P.B.

References

1 Tavassoli M, Crosby WH: Transplantation of marrow to extramedullary sites. Science 1968;161:54–56.

2 Friedenstein AJ: Precursor cells of mechanocytes. Int Rev Cytol 1976;47:327–359.

3 Friedenstein AJ: Stromal mechanisms of bone marrow: cloning in vitro and retransplantation in vivo. Hamatol Bluttransfus 1980;25:19–29.

4 Friedenstein AJ, Chailakhjan RK, Lalykina KS: The development of fibroblast colonies in monolayer cultures of guinea- pig bone marrow and spleen cells. Cell Tissue Kinet 1970;3:393–403.

5 Friedenstein AJ, Chailakhyan RK, Gerasimov UV: Bone marrow osteogenic stem cells: in vitro cultivation and transplantation in diffusion chambers. Cell Tissue Kinet 1987;20:263–272.

6 Friedenstein AJ, Latzinik NV, Gorskaya YF, Luria EA, Moskvina IL: Bone marrow stromal colony formation requires stimulation by haemopoietic cells. Bone Miner 1992;18:199–213.

7 Friedenstein AJ, Piatetzky-Shapiro II, Petrakova KV: Osteogenesis in transplants of bone marrow cells. J Embryol Exp Morphol 1966;16:381–390.

8 Friedenstein AJ: Osteogenic stem cells in bone marrow; in Heersche JNM, Kanis JA (eds): Bone and Mineral Research. Amsterdam, Elsevier, 1990.

9 Owen M, Friedenstein AJ: Stromal stem cells: marrow-derived osteogenic precursors. Ciba Found Symp 1988;136:42–60.

10 Spangrude GJ, Heimfeld S, Weissman IL: Purification and characterization of mouse hematopoietic stem cells. Science 1988;241:58–62.

11 Osawa M, Hanada K, Hamada H, Nakauchi H: Long-term lymphohematopoietic reconstitution by a single CD34-low/negative hematopoietic stem cell. Science 1996;273:242–245.

12 Simmons PJ, Torok-Storb B: Identification of stromal cell precursors in human bone marrow by a novel monoclonal antibody, STRO-1. Blood 1991; 78:55–62.

13 Sacchetti B, Funari A, Michienzi S, et al: Self-renewing osteoprogenitors in bone marrow sinusoids can organize a hematopoietic microenvironment. Cell 2007;131:324–336.

14 Weiss L: The hematopoietic microenvironment of the bone marrow: an ultrastructural study of the stroma in rats. Anat Rec 1976;186:161–184.

15 Westen H, Bainton DF: Association of alkaline phosphatase-positive reticulum cells in bone marrow with granulocytic precursors. J Exp Med 1979; 150:919–937.

16 Bianco P, Boyde A: Confocal images of marrow stromal (Westen-Bainton) cells. Histochemistry 1993;100:93–99.

17 Shih IM: The role of CD146 (Mel-CAM) in biology and pathology. J Pathol 1999;189:4–11.

18 Bianco P, Robey PG, Simmons PJ: Mesenchymal stem cells: revisiting history, concepts, and assays. Cell Stem Cell 2008;2:313–319.

19 Caplan AI: Mesenchymal stem cells. J Orthop Res 1991;9:641–650.

20 Pittenger MF, Mackay AM, Beck SC, et al: Multilineage potential of adult human mesenchymal stem cells. Science 1999;284:143–147.

21 Crisan M, Yap S, Casteilla L, et al: A perivascular origin for mesenchymal stem cells in multiple human organs. Cell Stem Cell 2008;3:301–313.

22 Bianco P, Robey PG: Skeletal stem cells: in Lanza RP (ed): Handbook of Adult and Fetal Stem Cells. San Diego, Academic Press, 2004, pp 415–424.

23 Bianco P, Kuznetsov SA, Riminucci M, Gehron RP: Postnatal skeletal stem cells. Methods Enzymol 2006;419:117–148.

24 Friedenstein AJ, Chailakhyan RK, Latsinik NV, Panasyuk AF, Keiliss-Borok IV: Stromal cells responsible for transferring the microenvironment of the hemopoietic tissues. Cloning in vitro and retransplantation in vivo. Transplantation 1974;17: 331–340.

25 Chailakhyan RK, Gerasimov IV, Fridenshtein A: Transfer of bone marrow microenvironment by clones of stromal mechanocytes. Bull Exper Biol Med 1978;86:1633–1635.

26 Kuznetsov SA, Krebsbach PH, Satomura K, et al: Single-colony derived strains of human marrow stromal fibroblasts form bone after transplantation in vivo. J Bone Miner Res 1997;12:1335–1347.

27 Calvi LM, Adams GB, Weibrecht KW, et al: Osteoblastic cells regulate the haematopoietic stem cell niche. Nature 2003;425:841–846.

28 Zhang J, Niu C, Ye L, et al: Identification of the haematopoietic stem cell niche and control of the niche size. Nature 2003;425:836–841.

29 Kiel MJ, Yilmaz OH, Iwashita T, Terhorst C, Morrison SJ: SLAM family receptors distinguish hematopoietic stem and progenitor cells and reveal endothelial niches for stem cells. Cell 2005;121:1109–1121.

30 Moore KA, Lemischka IR: Stem cells and their niches. Science 2006;311:1880–1885.

31 Morrison SJ, Spradling AC: Stem cells and niches: mechanisms that promote stem cell maintenance throughout life. Cell 2008;132:598–611.

32 Scadden DT: The stem cell niche in health and leukemic disease. Best Pract Res Clin Haematol 2007; 20:19–27.

33 Bianco P, Robey P: Diseases of bone and the stromal cell lineage. J Bone Miner Res 1999;14:336–341.

34 Bianco P, Robey PG: Marrow stromal stem cells. J Clin Invest 2000;105:1663–1668.

35 Holmbeck K, Bianco P, Chrysovergis K, Yamada S, Birkedal-Hansen H: MT1-MMP-dependent, apoptotic remodeling of unmineralized cartilage: a critical process in skeletal growth. J Cell Biol 2003; 163:661–671.

36 Bianco P, Riminucci M, Kuznetsov S, Robey PG: Multipotential cells in the bone marrow stroma: regulation in the context of organ physiology. Crit Rev Eukaryot Gene Expr 1999;9:159–173.

37 Calvi LM, Sims NA, Hunzelman JL, et al: Activated parathyroid hormone/parathyroid hormone-related protein receptor in osteoblastic cells differentially affects cortical and trabecular bone. J Clin Invest 2001;107:277–286.

38 Kuznetsov SA, Riminucci M, Ziran N, et al: The interplay of osteogenesis and hematopoiesis: expression of a constitutively active PTH/PTHrP receptor in osteogenic cells perturbs the establishment of hematopoiesis in bone and of skeletal stem cells in the bone marrow. J Cell Biol 2004;167:1113–1122.

39 Krebsbach PH, Kuznetsov SA, Satomura K, Emmons RV, Rowe DW, Robey PG: Bone formation in vivo: comparison of osteogenesis by transplanted mouse and human marrow stromal fibroblasts. Transplantation 1997;63:1059–1069.

40 Antonelli-Orlidge A, Saunders KB, Smith SR, D'Amore PA: An activated form of transforming growth factor beta is produced by cocultures of endothelial cells and pericytes. Proc Natl Acad Sci USA 1989;86:4544–4548.

41 Arai F, Hirao A, Ohmura M, et al: Tie2/angiopoietin-1 signaling regulates hematopoietic stem cell quiescence in the bone marrow niche. Cell 2004;118: 149–161.

42 Jain RK: Molecular regulation of vessel maturation. Nat Med 2003;9:685–693.

43 Satomura K, Krebsbach P, Bianco P, Gehron Robey P: Osteogenic imprinting upstream of marrow stromal cell differentiation. J Cell Biochem 2000;78: 391–403.

44 Bianco P, Robey PG: Stem cells in tissue engineering. Nature 2001;414:118–121.

45 Bianco P, Gehron Robey P, Wientroub S: Fibrous dysplasia; in Glorieux FH Pettifor JM, Jüppner H (ed): Pediatric Bone. Amsterdam, Elsevier 2003, pp 509–539.

46 Riminucci M, Fisher LW, Shenker A, Spiegel AM, Bianco P, Gehron Robey P: Fibrous dysplasia of bone in the McCune-Albright syndrome: abnormalities in bone formation. Am J Pathol 1997;151: 1587–1600.

47 Riminucci M, Liu B, Corsi A, et al: The histopathology of fibrous dysplasia of bone in patients with activating mutations of the Gs alpha gene: site-specific patterns and recurrent histological hallmarks. J Pathol 1999;187:249–258.

48 Bianco P, Kuznetsov SA, Riminucci M, Fisher LW, Spiegel AM, Robey PG: Reproduction of human fibrous dysplasia of bone in immunocompromised mice by transplanted mosaics of normal and Gsalpha-mutated skeletal progenitor cells. J Clin Invest 1998;101:1737–1744.
49 Riminucci M, Saggio I, Gehron Robey P, Bianco P: Fibrous dysplasia as a stem cell disease. J Bone Miner Res 2006;21(suppl 2):P125–P131.
50 Riminucci M, Collins MT, Fedarko NS, et al: FGF-23 in fibrous dysplasia of bone and its relationship to renal phosphate wasting. J Clin Invest 2003; 112:683–692.
51 Kuznetsov SA, Cherman N, Riminucci M, Collins MT, Robey PG, Bianco P: Age-dependent demise of GNAS-mutated skeletal stem cells and 'normalization' of fibrous dysplasia of bone. J Bone Miner Res 2008;23:1731–1740.
52 Piersanti S, Remoli C, Saggio I, et al: Transfer, analysis, and reversion of the fibrous dysplasia cellular phenotype in human skeletal progenitors. J Bone Miner Res 2010;25:1103–1116.

Prof. Paolo Bianco
Department of Molecular Medicine, Division of Pathology, Sapienza University of Rome
Viale Regina Elena 324
IT–00161 Rome (Italy)
Tel. +39 06 444 1049, E-Mail paolo.bianco@uniroma1.it

Camacho-Hübner C, Nilsson O, Sävendahl L (eds): Cartilage and Bone Development and Its Disorders.
Endocr Dev. Basel, Karger, 2011, vol 21, pp 102–115

Cartilage Tissue Engineering

Liliana S. Moreira-Teixeira · Nicole Georgi · Jeroen Leijten · Ling Wu · Marcel Karperien

Department of Tissue Regeneration, MIRA Institute for Biomedical Technology and Technical Medicine, University of Twente, Enschede, The Netherlands

Abstract

Cartilage tissue engineering is the art aimed at repairing defects in the articular cartilage which covers the bony ends in the joints. Since its introduction in the early 1990s of the past century, cartilage tissue engineering using ACI has been used in thousands of patients to repair articular cartilage defects. This review focuses on emerging strategies to improve cartilage repair by incorporating fundamental knowledge of developmental and cell biology in the design of optimized strategies for cell delivery at the defect site and to locally stimulate cartilage repair responses.

Tissue engineering is the art of utilizing (biological) material to generate a new tissue that will replace worn out or lost native tissue that mimics its original function. Mature joint cartilage is unable to repair itself sufficiently when damaged. This results in degeneration of the cartilage and inevitably joint failure. The need to intervene in this progressive degeneration and to restore or replace the affected cartilage effectively has created the field of cartilage tissue engineering. The main aim of cartilage tissue engineering is to repair joint or articular cartilage. Like epiphyseal growth plate cartilage, articular cartilage is a hyaline cartilage of which the ECM is rich in glycosaminoglycans and collagen type 2 as the most abundant protein. Unlike for articular cartilage, there is no clear clinical need for epiphyseal cartilage tissue engineering. Thus, if one speaks about cartilage tissue engineering, we are specifically talking about articular cartilage.

This review first discusses the development of cartilage focusing on the development of long bones, the growth plate and in particular articular cartilage. Many of the molecular mechanisms identified in the developing long bones can be applied

L.S.M.-T., N.G. and J.L. made equal contributions to this work.

in tissue engineering strategies. In addition to the biological knowledge, it is important to understand the history of clinical applications of articular cartilage repair and how this led to presently used tissue engineering strategies. Another essential element for the creation of an optimal and effective therapy is, in case cells are used, the cell source. For this the focus will be on historically used cell sources, the current trend and options for future therapy. The use of currently available commercial biomaterials and their use in cartilage tissue engineering, as well as emerging smart materials that are adapted to certain selected requirements are highlighted. Finally, this review gives a perspective on the future of cartilage tissue engineering.

Development of Cartilage

Joint Formation

The main purpose of tissue engineering is to generate new tissue that can mimic the original functions to replace worn out or lost native tissues. Fundamental knowledge on the tissue of interest, as well as its natural development, is therefore of paramount importance. Chondrogenesis is heralded from three different origins: the cranial neural crest that forms craniofacial cartilage, the somites leading to the axial skeleton and the lateral plate mesoderm resulting in the formation of limbs. From here on, we will focus on the latter, since cartilage tissue engineering mostly focuses on the joints of the limbs [1].

Secretion of FGF7 from the lateral plate mesoderm initiates the formation of the limb organizing apical ectodermal ridge. Subsequently, a signaling loop between FGF10 in the limb mesoderm and FGF8 in the apical ectodermal ridge directs the proximal distal outgrowth of the limb buds. Cartilage formation starts with the mesenchymal condensations in these developing limb buds and is formed from a seemingly heterogeneous cell population. The upregulation of TGF-β, a member of the BMP superfamily, leads to enhanced expression of numerous molecules including N-cadherin, N-CAM, fibronectin and tenascin-C, which are all implicated in the condensation of the mesenchymal cells [2].

Initiation of the expression of the cartilage master regulator SOX9 instigates chondrogenesis and is associated with the expression of collagen type IIA and at a later stage its splice variant collagen type IIB. Under the influence of a growth factor cocktail, including amongst others insulin growth factor-1, FGF2 and BMPs 2, 4, 7 and 14, the mesenchymal condensation develops into a cartilage anlage.

The determination of the location of the joint is dependent on a site called the interzone. Although the mechanism behind this phenomenon is largely unknown, the involvement of several molecules such as Wnt-14, GDF-5 and chordin has been implicated. The cells in the interzone start producing lubricin, which is suggested to play a role in the cavitation and separation of the original cartilage anlage resulting in the formation of the joint itself [3]. When fully formed, the articulated ends of the joints are still lined with lubricin-producing cells that will allow almost frictionless movement. In the mid-section of the remaining cartilage anlage, the primary center starts to mineralize and is eventually replaced by bone in a process called endochondral ossification. Postnatally, a second center of ossification appears in the primary growth plate that effectively separates the articular cartilage covering the distal ends of the long bone from the epiphyseal growth plate cartilage entrapped between the epiphysis and metaphysis. Unlike epiphyseal growth plate cartilage which disappears at the end of puberty by growth plate fusion, healthy articular cartilage is resistant to endochondral ossification and does not disappear after puberty.

Growth Plate Cartilage

Being primarily responsible for longitudinal growth, the activity of the epiphyseal growth plate is tightly orchestrated by multiple autocrine, paracrine and endocrine factors. After the initial mesenchymal condensation and chondrogenic differentiation, the chondrocytes in the center of the cartilage anlage start to undergo hypertrophic differentiation. This terminal differentiation allows for the formation of a mineralized matrix, in growth of blood vessels and eventually chondrocyte death, most likely via apoptosis. On the remaining cartilage anlage, osteoblasts start producing bone, forming the primary spongiosa. At the opposing end of the hypertrophic chondrocytes, chondrocyte proliferation continues in vertical columns further lengthening the long bones. These proliferating chondrocytes are recruited from the resting zone which covers the distal ends of the long bones. After the formation of the secondary ossification center, the resting zone is located directly adjacent to the epiphysis [4] and contains the growth plate stem cells. The continuous cycle of stem cell recruitment, proliferation, hypertrophic differentiation and chondrocyte death is tightly regulated by a plethora of signaling molecules. The feedback loop between IHH and PTHrP is demonstrated to be one of the key regulators of endochondral ossification. Additionally, many other factors have been shown to play (major) roles in endochondral ossification including paracrine factors like FGFs, BMPs, WNTs, and endocrine regulators such as thyroid hormone, GH, IGF-I, testosterone and estrogens [5]. Many of these factors are currently explored for application in tissue engineering strategies for cartilage repair.

Articular Cartilage

As already indicated, the main focus of cartilage tissue engineering is on restoration of the articulated surface of the joint, the articular cartilage. In its healthy mature form, the tissue has an extremely high matrix/cell ratio: only 2–3% of its mass consists of chondrocytes, the only residing cells in articular cartilage. For the remaining, 65–80% consists of water, 12–21% of collagens being predominantly collagen type II, 6–10% of proteoglycans and approximately 2–3.5% other proteins. The arch-like orientation of collagen type II fibrils, being almost horizontal in the superficial zone and almost fully vertical in the deep zone, gives the articular cartilage its anisotropic nature and allows it to transduce mechanical forces throughout the entire tissue. Additionally, the different zones do not contain the same (ratio of) molecules, having different (levels of) glycosaminoglycans and collagens as well as other more characteristic features such as the calcification of the cartilage near the subchondral bone and the production of lubricin in the superficial zone [6]. An important characteristic of healthy articular cartilage is that it is resistant to endochondral ossification. In joint degenerative diseases such as osteoarthritis, this resistance disappears, and it is described that the degeneration is, at least in part, caused by endochondral ossification [7]. Articular and epiphyseal chondrocytes have many features in common, and it has long been believed that they have a common progenitor. In the past years, however, preliminary proof has been provided that articular and epiphyseal growth plate chondrocytes arise from distinct cell populations. At present, the mechanisms by which articular chondrocytes are formed and by which they are able to resist hypertrophic differentiation and subsequent endochondral ossification remains unknown.

History of Clinical Applications in Cartilage Repair

The clinical and biological need to develop new cartilage repair strategies arises from the fact that cartilage has a low capacity of self-repair. When damaged by either trauma or degenerative diseases, it will progressively degrade and thereby destabilize the joint. The majority of cartilage engineering strategies focus on the repair of cartilage lesions induced by trauma, since progressively diseased cartilage, such as seen in osteoarthritis needs different repair approach.

If left untreated, acute trauma will inevitably result in joint degeneration necessitating unicompartmental or total joint replacement as the only possible solution to treat the degenerated joint. To avoid total joint replacement, the surgeon has a number of treatment options, all with inherent drawbacks. The most popular clinical cartilage repair approaches of the last 20 years are osteochondral transplantation, marrow stimulation techniques, e.g. MF and ACI.

Osteochondral transplantation can be divided into autologous mosaicplasty and allograft osteochondral transplantation. In the more recently developed mosaicplasty [8], cylindrical osteochondral grafts are harvested from a non-load-bearing site of the donor and will then be press fitted in pre-drilled osteochondral holes of the defect area. During the healing process, the space between the grafts will be filled with fibrocartilaginous tissue. This strategy carries the risk of bone collapse at the donor and recipient site, but shows acceptable results in long-term follow-up. Since mosaicplasty can only be applied to smaller lesions, allograft osteochondral transplantation with matching fresh or frozen cartilage pieces from organ donors is an alternative option.

During MF, the subchondral bone of the affected cartilage is perforated leading to blood clot formation at the defect site and, after the invasion of progenitor cells, to cartilage matrix formation. This cost saving and fast technique, based on the self-

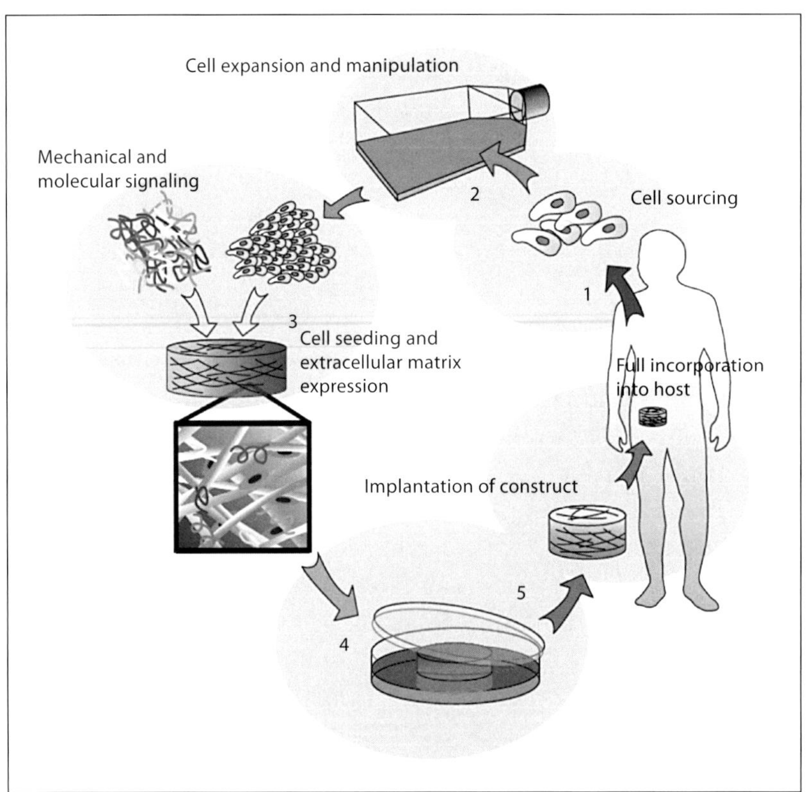

Fig. 1. The tissue engineering approach. Adapted from van Blitterswijk [27].

healing capacity of invading bone marrow cells, was first introduced by Steadman et al. [9] in the early 1990s. The procedure of MF leads to satisfactory outcome, but has been reported to induce fibrous cartilage formation with poor mechanical properties in some cases, questioning the long-term performance of the de novo formed tissue. Next to MF, ACI gained popularity after its introduction by Brittberg et al. [10] in 1994. ACI is the first cell-based therapeutic cartilage tissue engineering strategy. This two-step surgical procedure requires donor cartilage harvest from a non-load-bearing site for chondrocyte isolation, followed by up to 6 weeks of cell expansion ex vivo and finally reimplantation of the expanded cells at the defect site. During reimplantation, the cartilage defect is first covered with a periosteal flap sealed with fibrin glue before injecting the cultured chondrocytes underneath the periosteal flap (fig. 1). This time-consuming and costly technique has been shown to promote the formation of hyaline like cartilage with functional improvement in most patients, whereas other studies provide evidence for the abundance of substantial amounts of fibrous cartilage [11]. In the last decade, various studies compared MF with ACI with conflicting results. The findings indicate that ACI and MF lead to similar outcomes in the repair of small lesions, but the repair of large defects might have a superior outcome after

ACI. In 2008, Saris et al. [12] introduced characterized chondrocyte implantation to overcome existing problems with the quality of the engineered cartilage obtained by ACI. The strategy of this characterized chondrocyte implantation relies on the preassessment of chondrocyte populations with a greater potential to form hyaline cartilage. Compared with MF, this technique was shown to result in noticeably better clinical outcome after 36 months [13].

Although all these described cartilage repair strategies support enhanced joint function and pain relief for the patient, they do not succeed in restoring the natural cartilage structure with its associated biomechanical properties. Recent cartilage tissue engineering approaches include established methods in combination with the delivery of cells and/or bioactive molecules via a biomaterial scaffold. Bartlett and colleagues described two variations of the traditional ACI. In the first variation, periosteal flap is replaced with a porcine-derived type I/type III collagen (ACI-C) matrix. In the second variation, before implantation chondrocytes were first seeded in a collagen bilayer (matrix-induced ACI). Both methods resulted in an improvement of ACI based on the Cincinnati knee score and International Cartilage Repair Society score, which provide both a measure for cartilage and joint quality.

Cell Sources of Cartilage Engineering

Presently, cartilage tissue engineering is primarily based on the use of two cell types: chondrocytes or MSCs. As the most intuitive cell source for cartilage regeneration, autologous chondrocytes have been successfully used in many studies of cartilage repair with or without the use of a scaffold [10]. However, using chondrocytes in cartilage repair applications obviously has some disadvantages. One problem could be injury of healthy cartilage from which chondrocytes are harvested. Although donor cartilage is taken from low weight-bearing sites of joint, this procedure often results in morbidity at donor sites. Another problem of using autologous chondrocytes in cartilage engineering is that they can only be harvested from small biopsies of articular cartilage. To obtain sufficient chondrocytes for cartilage repair, in vitro expansion is necessary. Culture expansion of chondrocytes results in a gradual loss of the chondrocyte phenotype with increasing passage number, a process known as chondrocyte dedifferentiation.

After several passages of expansion in two-dimensional culture environment, chondrocytes lose their initial characteristics and become fibroblast-like cells [14]. Expanding chondrocytes on microcarriers instead of tissue culture plastic can omit subculture steps in flask, thus preventing dedifferentiation of chondrocytes. It is also believed that dedifferentiated chondrocytes may regain the ability to produce cartilage matrix when cultured in a 3-D environment (e.g. suspension in hydro-gel), or in chondrogenic differentiation medium containing TFG-β. This growth factor plays an important role in cartilage formation during organogenesis in the embryo. However, the cartilage phenotypes obtained by these treatments are significantly inferior when compared to native cartilage [15]. Yet, the complex molecular events occurring in the induction and maintenance of the chondrogenic phenotype should still be enlightened for further identification of the bioactive levels and kinetics of the key factors involved in cartilage repair. Moreover, integration of repair cartilage with the native tissue and reestablishment of the zonal organization of articular cartilage are still challenging and only partly resolved.

To improve the quantity of regenerated cartilage, MSCs are considered to be a promising alternative cell source. MSCs are adult stem cells isolated from somatic tissue. They have been found to be multipotent, showing the ability to differentiate into chondrocyte, osteoblast, adipocytes and endothelial cells. MSCs isolated from different origins like bone marrow, fat tissue, synovium and muscles all show potency of chondrogenic differentiation, and may have possible applications in cartilage tissue engineering [16]. Most clinical studies use autologous MSCs, though allograft MSCs may be used in some cases. Traditionally, ex vivo chondrogenic differentiation of MSCs is induced by culturing high-density cell pellets in serum-free medium containing TGF-β. High-density pellets mimic the first step of cartilage formation in the embryo, namely the condensation of mesenchymal cells. For MSCs isolated from fat tissue, BMP-6 is often added to the differentiation medium. In recent years, it has been reported that culturing MSCs in gel-like biomaterials made of collagen or fibrin increases chondrogenic differentiation of MSCs when compared with pellet culture [17]. When using MSCs for cartilage engineering, the greatest challenge is not the differentiation of the cells into chondrocytes per se but to prevent the chondrogenically differentiated MSCs from undergoing endochondral ossification. Substantial evidence indicates that the chondrogenically differentiated MSCs acquire an epiphyseal growth plate phenotype rather than an articular phenotype [18]. To direct differentiation of MSCs into the articular cartilage lineage instead of a growth plate lineage is an active area of research.

To reduce the number of chondrocytes needed for cartilage engineering, MSCs started to be cocultured with chondrocytes. Interestingly, it was reported that cocultures of bone marrow MSCs with articular chondrocytes produced more matrix compared to chondrocytes alone [19]. This phenomenon of increased cartilage formation was not only observed in differentiation medium containing TGF-β, but also in medium without any growth factors. Enhancement of cartilage matrix formation was also found in cocultures of articular chondrocytes with other sources of MSCs [20]. This effect has been attributed to the chondrogenic differentiation of MSCs stimulated by the chondrocytes. In recent years, it has been suggested that lineage commitment of MSCs cannot fully explain their benefits on tissue remodeling and repair. Many studies have suggested a role for MSCs in secreting trophic mediators that stimulate local tissue repair mechanisms. These factors promote tissue-specific cells to restore the damaged or lost tissue. A combination of MSCs and autologous chondrocytes may be a promising strategy for cartilage engineering in which the trophic effects of MSCs support and facilitate the chondrocytes to repair cartilage defects. The strategy also reveals possibility of omitting in vitro expansion of chondrocytes in traditional ACI procedures. The mixture of chondrocyte and MSCs may lead to a single step surgery for cartilage treatment, in which chondrocytes are isolated, mixed with bone marrow cells from the same patient, loaded on a scaffold and directly reimplanted into the patient.

Many aspects of ACI still need further optimization. For example, the integration of the neo tissue is still far from optimal. It can be hindered by cell loss, either by apoptosis or necrosis caused by, for example, inflammatory cytokines or mechanical stress, or due to leakage of the cells. The relatively limited ECM production by the implanted cells, and the dissimilarities in structure and/or composition compared to native cartilage can also lead to integration failure. Thus, strategies that circumvent these complex molecular events, such as the delivery of anti-apoptotic or anti-dedifferentiating factors, combined with a structural orchestration of cells and soluble factors, are thought to play an essential role in future therapies.

Biomaterials for Cartilage Repair

The commonly used strategy of tissue engineering is, in general terms, to seed cells in a scaffold that can be implanted into the damaged site, as illustrated in figure 1. Initially, the main purpose of the scaffold is to provide structural support and allow attachment, proliferation and differentiation of cells in a 3-D environment. The mechanical support provided by the scaffold would lead to a decrease in the rehabilitation time for the patient. Nowadays, tissue engineered scaffolds may be developed to trigger, interact and instruct cells by mimicry of key molecular features of the native ECM, conferred by both macromolecules (proteoglycans, collagens, fibronectin and laminins) and sequestered growth factors [21].

Chondro-Conducting Scaffolds: Natural and Synthetic Biomaterials

A myriad of biomaterials has been used as scaffolds for 3-D culture of chondrocytes in vitro and in vivo, as well as for medical applications. Scaffolds can vary depending on material chemistry, 3-D geometry, structure, mechanical properties and speed of degradation. The structure, mainly described in terms of pore distribution, orientation and connectivity, should maximize exchange of nutrients, metabolites and regulatory factors, as well as limit oxygen gradients and influence cell-cell interactions. The chemistry can play an instructional role and, overall, the scaffold should be biocompatible and biodegrade at a similar rate as ECM deposition to ensure continuity and stability of the neo-tissue [22]. Additionally, the scaffolds' mechanical integrity and integration should not only be sufficient to support

Table 1. Scaffold materials for cartilage repair

Material source	Examples	Advantages/disadvantages
Natural	Collagen based	Advantage: providers of molecular cues to the cells, stimulating them to produce more collagen. Disadvantage: poor mechanical properties and can undergo contraction due to interactions with cells when not combined with other materials.
	Hyaluronic acid	Advantage: bioactive properties, with the ability of interacting with chondrocytes (via CD44). Disadvantage: poor mechanical properties of the unmodified hyaluronic acid; the combination or engraftment with other materials, such as polyethylene glycol or dextran, allowed optimization of the biomechanical properties of the hyaluronic acid-based scaffolds.
	Fibrin glue	Advantage: extensively used for wound healing and, additionally for its use as fixative for scaffolds to native tissue. It can also be used as a matrix. Disadvantage: enhancement of cartilage repair is limited.
	Chitosan, agarose and alginate	Advantage: used as either hydrogels, sponges or pads. Disadvantage: still not available for clinical applications.
Synthetic	Polylactide, polyglycolide, polyethylene glycol and polyurethane	Advantage: no batch variation. Disadvantage: possible inflammatory response against degradation products.

or match the native tissue, but also mediate mechanical stimulus to the cells during loading [23].

Scaffold materials for cartilage repair can be distinguished according to their source: natural or synthetic, as shown in table 1. Natural biomaterials can also be divided into two types: protein and polysaccharide based. Many of these natural materials can be degraded by human enzymes, with nontoxic degradation products. Yet, these materials have some drawbacks, mainly related to batch variation, processing and potential pathogen transfer. The main natural materials used for cartilage tissue engineering are collagen, hyaluronic acid, chitosan, agarose, alginate and fibrin glue [24]. These materials can be used either as temporary scaffolds and/or vehicles for cell and drug delivery or can be directly implanted or injected into the defect site.

Synthetic polymers are widely used in tissue engineering due to their flexibility in design and absence of the possibility of disease transmission; yet the disadvantages

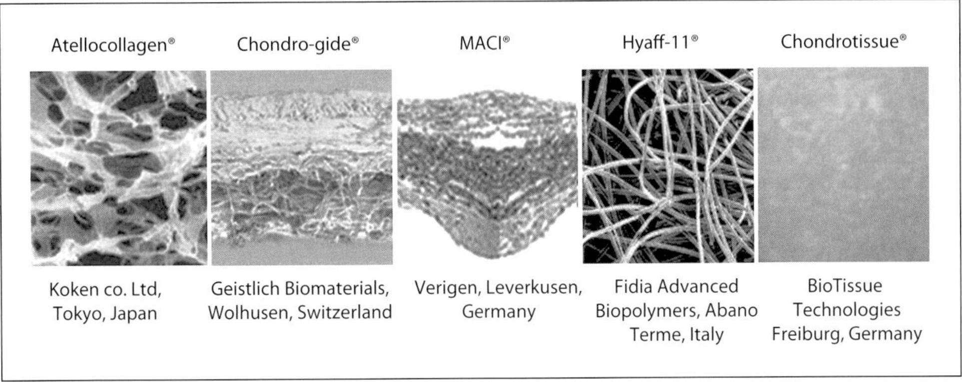

Fig. 2. Protein-based membranes and gels already available for ACI.

are related to their relatively poor biocompatibility, for example of degradation products, which can lead to severe inflammatory responses. Synthetic materials, such as polylactide, polyglycolide and polyurethane, have been explored as suitable candidates for cartilage repair [24]. Figure 2 shows some protein-based membranes and gels which are currently explored in ACI procedures.

Scaffolds developed for cartilage tissue engineering can be either solid, like foam meshes or sponges, or gel-like, also termed as hydrogels. Hydrogels have been largely explored for cartilage repair strategies, because they consist of 3-D hydrophilic networks and their high water content mimics native cartilage, unlike solid-type materials. Additionally, due to high diffusion rates, hydrogels allow efficient transport of nutrients and waste products. Hydrogels can be composed of natural and/or synthetic polymers that form a gellified network by physical, ionic or covalent crosslinking. Some hydrogels can be thermo-reversible (liquid at approximately 25°C or below, only solidifying at body temperature, around 37°C) or crosslinked, either chemically (for example by enzymes), or by photo-polymerization (using visible or ultraviolet light). In situ forming hydrogels allow for replacement of open surgeries by a minimal invasive procedure that offers great advantages in integration with native tissue and limits the trauma caused by surgery.

Emerging 'Smart' Biomaterials

Novel scaffolds based on modification of natural polymers, such as dextran, silk, heparin and cellulose, or of synthetic polymers, such as polycaprolactone or copolymers of polyether-esters have been studied to support cartilage regeneration. Several of these studies have focused on the optimization of these materials and have shown that the combination of different materials may improve properties [24]. Hybrid materials can be designed to mimic ECM structure, for example by adding hyaluronic acid or chondroitin-6-sulfate, and, therefore, providing direct interaction with the chondrocytes by enabling the necessary signals to trigger tissue repair. The communication between the cells and ECM can also be mediated by integrins, surface-specific receptors that react with proteins, such as collagens, fibronectin and laminin, which affect cell survival, proliferation and differentiation. To facilitate these types of interactions, short synthetic peptides such as the Arg-Gly-Asp (RGD) sequence, can be incorporated into scaffolds to increase the interaction between biomaterials and cells. These recognition sequences have proven to be of great value in the case of synthetic materials that lack cell attachment signals. Yet, the involvement of the RGD sequence in inducing or supporting chondrogenic differentiation of MSCs is still controversial. In addition to these peptides, the controlled local delivery of growth and differentiation factors, including IGF-I, TGF-β_1 and TGF-β_3 or BMP-2 and BMP-6, has been successfully combined with scaffolds. These growth factors have been selected based on their proven role during cartilogenesis in the developing embryo. Hybrid scaffolds can either be designed to locally release the bioactive factors or produced in such a way that they mimic properties of the ECM. The release of growth factors by synthetic polymers is still highly dependent on the diffusion and degradation rates of the polymers.

Recently, surface-eroding scaffolds and materials of which the release occurs by cellular demand have been developed to allow a better and more effective control of the release profiles. By incorporation in the scaffold of peptide sequences which can be recognized by e.g. MMPs, release of growth factors can be locally controlled [25]. This responsive feature of the scaffold can be of great interest as the release of the growth factor in these cases can be tailored to depend on the disease activity. For example, MMP-13 is a factor that is significantly elevated in osteoarthritis and can be used as a trigger to release scaffold-bound drugs [24].

Other strategies to improve scaffold design include the development of biphasic scaffolds. Such scaffolds can also be used in vitro for tissue formation prior to implantation, where the design prevents cell migration between regions of the scaffold [23]. Like the growth plate, articular cartilage has a zonal organization. Strategies have been developed that use predefined geometries (for example by using rapid prototyping technologies), or have incorporated physical and chemical gradients in the scaffold to recreate the zonal organization in tissue-engineered constructs [26]. Using these strategies, the mimicry of the native cartilage-tissue anisotropy can be achieved. Gene therapy approaches can also be taken into account in scaffold design. In recent years, promising results for cartilage repair strategies have been obtained by transfecting chondro-generative growth factor genes and/or chondro-protective cartilage catabolic inhibitor genes [23].

Starting from structural variations from nano- to macroscale, the new generation of scaffolds often with a bioinspired design, aim at creating the optimal microenvironment for the formation of a de novo extracellular cartilaginous matrix by either chondrocytes, MSCs or a combination of both cell types.

Future of Cartilage Tissue Engineering

Although a wide range of possible cartilage repair strategies have been described, none of them successfully restores the function and organization of cartilage in long-term studies. At the moment, numerous possible novel repair strategies arise. In general, the optimal approach will be determined by three major components: cells, biomaterials and bioactive compounds.

Cellular and molecular studies including improved cell culture, coculture, cell tracking, gene therapy, gene arrays and proteomics will provide further cues for possible strategies in joint surface regeneration. The complex molecular events occurring in the induction and maintenance of the chondrogenic phenotype during embryogenesis may lead to the identification of novel mechanisms involved in cartilage formation. It seems promising to translate the findings from developmental biology into strategies for cartilage tissue formation. Apart from optimized allogenic and autologous cartilage or cell transplants, progenitor cells, like autologous bone marrow-derived stromal cells (MSCs), are likely to play an important role in future strategies for cartilage tissue repair being an alternative or supplementary cell source. Until now, however, the fate of these cells, the choice of cell fraction and optimal culture parameters are not determined, and additional research is needed to clarify their applicability to articular cartilage engineering.

As indicated above, growth factors may play an important role in further optimization of cartilage tissue engineering. Presently, application of growth factors in cartilage tissue engineering is controversial, and more robust studies are needed to demonstrate their applicability. The choice of the optimal combination of growth factor and method of delivery will very likely depend on the cell type used. For example, different growth factors may be needed when MSCs or expanded primary chondrocytes are used for cartilage repair. Improvements in growth factor delivery should reflect an extended release profile, with protection of the proteins against fast degradation, and must aim at targeting specific cell types. Multistep release, as a polytherapy approach instead of single delivery systems, could be an additional improvement for cartilage repair strategies.

The third pillar of cartilage tissue engineering is formed by biomaterials. At the moment, evermore biomaterials are being developed that show better bioaffinity and manage to mimic the native environment of cartilage. An example of these new generations of biomaterials are in situ gelating hydrogels, which mimic the natural ECM and can perfectly fill up irregular defect sites. Importantly, in situ gelating hydrogels can be used in minimal invasive strategies, which will significantly reduce the burden for the individual patient.

'Smart' hydrogels sensitive to external stimuli such as temperature, pH or certain biomolecules, that can trigger swelling or degradation, have been developed. Recently, dynamic hydrogels have been investigated, offering the ability to precisely control temporal and spatial behavior of the cells, by creating a tissue-like hierarchical organization. This strategy can be combined with tailored delivery of bioactive signals that stimulate tissue repair.

Translating fundamental knowledge of chondrogenesis and articular cartilage homeostasis into the design of novel smart materials is an active field of research which undoubtedly will result in the development of improved strategies for cartilage repair in the near future.

References

1 Olsen BR, Reginato AM, Wang W: Bone development. Annu Rev Cell Dev Biol 2000;16:191–220.

2 Chimal-Monroy J, Diaz de Leon L: Expression of N-cadherin, N-CAM, fibronectin and tenascin is stimulated by TGF-beta1, beta2, beta3 and beta5 during the formation of precartilage condensations. Int J Dev Biol 1999;43:59–67.

3 Pacifici M, Koyama E, Iwamoto M: Mechanisms of synovial joint and articular cartilage formation: recent advances, but many lingering mysteries. Birth Defects Res C Embryo Today 2005;75:237–248.

4 Zuscik MJ, Hilton MJ, Zhang X, Chen D, O'Keefe RJ: Regulation of chondrogenesis and chondrocyte differentiation by stress. J Clin Invest 2008;118:429–438.

5 Grumbach MM: Estrogen, bone, growth and sex: a sea change in conventional wisdom. J Pediatr Endocrinol Metab 2000;13(suppl 6):1439–1455.

6 Poole AR, Kojima T, Yasuda T, Mwale F, Kobayashi M, Laverty S: Composition and structure of articular cartilage: a template for tissue repair. Clin Orthop Relat Res 2001:S26–S33.

7 Kawaguchi H: Regulation of osteoarthritis development by Wnt-beta-catenin signaling through the endochondral ossification process. J Bone Miner Res 2009;24:8–11.

8 Hangody L, Kish G, Karpati Z, Szerb I, Udvarhelyi I: Arthroscopic autogenous osteochondral mosaicplasty for the treatment of femoral condylar articular defects. A preliminary report. Knee Surg Sports Traumatol Arthrosc 1997;5:262–267.

9 Steadman JR, Rodkey WG, Briggs KK, Rodrigo JJ: The microfracture technic in the management of complete cartilage defects in the knee joint (in German). Orthopade 1999;28:26–32.

10 Brittberg M, Lindahl A, Nilsson A, Ohlsson C, Isaksson O, Peterson L: Treatment of deep cartilage defects in the knee with autologous chondrocyte transplantation. N Engl J Med 1994;331:889–895.

11 McNickle AG, L'Heureux DR, Yanke AB, Cole BJ: Outcomes of autologous chondrocyte implantation in a diverse patient population. Am J Sports Med 2009;37:1344–1350.

12 Saris DB, Vanlauwe J, Victor J, et al: Characterized chondrocyte implantation results in better structural repair when treating symptomatic cartilage defects of the knee in a randomized controlled trial versus microfracture. Am J Sports Med 2008;36:235–246.

13 Saris DB, Vanlauwe J, Victor J, et al: Treatment of symptomatic cartilage defects of the knee: characterized chondrocyte implantation results in better clinical outcome at 36 months in a randomized trial compared to microfracture. Am J Sports Med 2009;37(suppl 1):10S–19S.

14 Schnabel M, Marlovits S, Eckhoff G, et al: Dedifferentiation-associated changes in morphology and gene expression in primary human articular chondrocytes in cell culture. Osteoarth Cartil 2002;10:62–70.

15 Mukaida T, Urabe K, Naruse K, et al: Influence of three-dimensional culture in a type II collagen sponge on primary cultured and dedifferentiated chondrocytes. J Orthop Sci 2005;10:521–528.

16 Sakaguchi Y, Sekiya I, Yagishita K, Muneta T: Comparison of human stem cells derived from various mesenchymal tissues: superiority of synovium as a cell source. Arthritis Rheum 2005;52:2521–2529.

17 Mueller MB, Tuan RS: Functional characterization of hypertrophy in chondrogenesis of human mesenchymal stem cells. Arthritis Rheum 2008;58:1377–1388.

18 Tsuchiya K, Chen GP, Ushida T, Matsuno T, Tateishi T: The effect of coculture of chondrocytes with mesenchymal stem cells on their cartilaginous phenotype in vitro. Mat Sci Eng C-Bio S 2004;24:391–396.

19 Hildner F, Concaro S, Peterbauer A, et al: Human adipose-derived stem cells contribute to chondrogenesis in coculture with human articular chondrocytes. Tissue Eng Pt A 2009;15:3961–3969.

20 Gnecchi M, He H, Liang OD, et al: Paracrine action accounts for marked protection of ischemic heart by Akt-modified mesenchymal stem cells. Nat Med 2005;11:367–368.
21 Place ES, Evans ND, Stevens MM: Complexity in biomaterials for tissue engineering. Nat Mater 2009;8:457–470.
22 Vunjak-Novakovic G: The fundamentals of tissue engineering: scaffolds and bioreactors. Novartis Found Symp 2003;249:34–46, discussion 46–51, 170–174, 239–241.
23 Woodfield TB, Bezemer JM, Pieper JS, van Blitterswijk CA, Riesle J: Scaffolds for tissue engineering of cartilage. Crit Rev Eukaryot Gene Expr 2002;12:209–236.
24 Stoop R: Smart biomaterials for tissue engineering of cartilage. Injury 2008;39(suppl 1):S77–S87.
25 Raeber GP, Lutolf MP, Hubbell JA: Mechanisms of 3-D migration and matrix remodeling of fibroblasts within artificial ECMs. Acta Biomater 2007;3:615–629.
26 Klein TJ, Malda J, Sah RL, Hutmacher DW: Tissue engineering of articular cartilage with biomimetic zones. Tissue Eng Part B Rev 2009;15:143–157.
27 van Blitterswijk CA: Tissue Engineering. Academic Press Series in Biomedical Engineering. Elsevier, Amsterdam/Academic Press, London, 2008, p 740.

Dr. Marcel Karperien
Department of Tissue Regeneration, MIRA Institute for Biomedical Technology and Technical Medicine, University of Twente
PO Box 217
NL–7500 AE Enschede (The Netherlands)
Tel. +31 53 489 3323, E-Mail h.b.j.karperien@tnw.utwente.nl

Author Index

Subject Index